PRIMARY NURSING
A MODEL FOR INDIVIDUALIZED CARE

PRIMARY NURSING

A MODEL FOR INDIVIDUALIZED CARE

GWEN D. MARRAM, R.N., Ph.D.

Chairman, Department of Nursing, San Jose State University,
San Jose, California

MARGARET W. SCHLEGEL, R.N.

Herrick Memorial Hospital, Berkeley, California

EM O. BEVIS, R.N., M.A.

Professor of Nursing, San Jose State University,
San Jose, California

with 23 illustrations

THE C. V. MOSBY COMPANY

SAINT LOUIS 1974

Library of Congress Cataloging in Publication Data

Marram, Gwen D   1942-
    Primary nursing.

    1.   Nurses and nursing.   I.   Schlegel, Margaret W.,
1941-   joint author.   II.   Bevis, Em Olivia, joint
author.   III.   Title.   [DNLM: 1. Nursing. 2. Nursing
care.   WY100 M358p 1974]
RT41.M37   610.73   73-20475
ISBN 0-8016-3128-9

GW/M/M   9   8   7   6   5   4   3   2

To   THE PATIENT

PREFACE

The organization of nursing care for the maximum benefit of patients and the maximum utilization and development of nurses is an onerous task. One would assume that high-quality nursing care and the maximum utilization of staff would go hand in hand. Still, in the everyday work world where nursing happens, we find that these ends are often miles apart if not blatantly conflicting. What has come to be the best utilization of staff can result in highly fragmented nursing care to patients. The problem then is to develop and implement a system that achieves the highest quality nursing care as well as an efficient means of delivering this care.

It has come to our attention and to the attention of our colleagues in health care agencies and schools of nursing that a text exploring the potentials of primary nursing is of vital importance to nurses in general and to those responsible for innovations in the nursing care delivery system. Unfortunately, such a text does not exist.

Primary Nursing is intended to fill this gap and thereby ease the adoption of primary nursing by caregiving groups. More specifically, the text discusses this approach to nursing care in depth and is explicit about the advantages of primary nursing over other existing nursing systems, the operationalization of primary nursing, and its effects on patients, physicians, and nursing staff. In addition, the text highlights several technological and professional trends that make primary nursing the most logical means of caring for patients and their families today.

This text is intended to benefit a rather broad audience in nursing, ranging from those students and clinicians giving direct nursing care to educators and administrators who are responsible for overseeing this innovation. Although the book may make its most significant contribution to nursing care in hospitals, clinicians in clinics and community health facilities will find it extremely useful. The text, together with opportunities to engage in supervised primary nursing experiences, will enhance the development of nurse clinicians and instill in them the ideals of sound, individualized patient care. In addition, it will deepen their understanding of the forces and contingencies that impend on the practice of nursing and dictate the organization of nursing care.

Although primary nursing is one of the most exciting innovations in the health care field, we use the term "innovation" with reservation. Perhaps we have come full circle in finding that, as before, the true role of the nurse is *giving* care as opposed to directing and supervising others. Nursing is still the primary function of nurses. In addition, it makes sense from the patient's point of view that the person responsible for his care should be the most knowledgeable about his unique needs as an individual.

This does not mean to imply that the nursing profession does not need more leaders. On the contrary, we need more leaders than ever before. From the efficiency viewpoint, it is also important that the skills and knowledge of the nurse still be transmitted to less knowledgeable members of the health team. Yet we must keep in mind that the most important function of the nurse is to continue to give and be held accountable for direct patient care. It is more than "getting back to the bedside" where the patient is; it is preserving and fostering ideal patient care, the one true value that nursing and only nursing can exercise to its utmost. In primary nursing the most important focal point is the patient and the quality of the care he receives. Directing and supervising others to do nursing takes its proper perspective, a function secondary to providing patients and their families with the best nursing care possible.

We have many to acknowledge for the ideas and inspiration expressed in this text. We would like to show gratitude to the many leaders in nursing across the country who took the time to respond to our surveys and inquiries. In particular, we wish to pay tribute to Marie Manthey, whose pioneering in the area of primary nursing gave us the inspiration to further "chart the territory."

Special thanks go to the administrators of hospitals in California and Iowa who made it possible to implement and experiment with different aspects of primary nursing. We are deeply indebted to the nursing staff at Merritt Hospital, Oakland, California, El Camino Hospital, Mt. View, California, and Iowa Methodist Medical Center, Des Moines, Iowa, who came up with plans for implementing primary nursing that do justice to the concept and caused their patients to exclaim with sincere gratitude: "I really feel that they care about me!"

Gwen D. Marram
Margaret W. Schlegel
Em O. Bevis

CONTENTS

INTRODUCTION

Because many new terms are used to describe modes of dispensing nursing care today, it is important to be aware of what is meant by "primary nursing" at the outset. Primary nursing as defined in this text is the distribution of nursing so that the total care of an individual patient is the responsibility of one nurse, not many nurses. Primary nursing can best be differentiated from team or functional nursing, which requires that the total care of any one patient be shared by several nurses during a single shift.

Primary nursing is more than a "new" way of organizing the delivery of nursing care. It implies a philosophy of nursing in which the patient is central to the focus of the nurse, and accountability of nurses for their patients is paramount.

Primary nursing also embodies a theoretical construct. It is a concept that includes prescriptions for the organization of nurses' work and as such generates propositions that can be grounded in experience and tested systematically as hypotheses. In this text we have collected several sets of data on hypotheses derived from the theory that primary nursing represents a distinct nursing modality that can be compared and contrasted with other nursing care modalities.

One of these propositions is that given a primary nursing system, patients will perceive their nursing care as highly individualized. Second, patients on a primary nursing care unit should more frequently describe their nursing care as highly unique to them as persons than patients on other units such as team nursing units.

It is important to note that all ways of organizing work lend themselves to experimentation, research, and evaluation. Unfortunately, nursing has been remiss in accepting its responsibility for establishing criteria and for testing the consequences of how nursing care is dispensed to clients and patients.

In this text a great deal of time is spent in placing primary nursing in a context, describing its operation, and exploring its results. These activities lay a foundation for systematic consideration and evaluation of this system compared to other systems.

Part I is devoted to the evaluation of modes of organizing nursing care of patients. The profession of nursing will be assessed in terms of its stages of development to shed light on how different care modalities arise, flourish, and subside in importance. Current factors that influence health care delivery will also be identified, illustrating the relationship between the profession, the imping-ing pressures to change, and nursing's reaction to respond by changes in ways of dispensing nursing care.

Part II deals with the nature and scope of primary nursing. It is here that we define in operational and concrete terms the minute operations of primary nurs-ing units. Primary nursing as employed in other settings across the country will be discussed. A model primary nursing unit will be described in detail for those interested in implementing primary nursing in their institutions. Organizational features that highlight and enhance coordination, continuity, and patient-centeredness in primary nursing will be outlined. Finally, the processes of change so necessary to innovation of this kind are identified and discussed.

The final section, Part III, will report the effects of primary nursing that we have found through our research to date. Outcomes for patients, effects on nurs-ing personnel, and attitudes of physicians and administrators will be discussed in separate chapters.

The text is summarized in Chapter 10, utilizing a question-answer format, in which we answer questions that occurred in consultation sessions with various administrators, physicians, and staff nurses across the country. These questions range in scope from what we think about the role of the head nurse on a primary nursing unit to what we are suggesting about the function of nursing education, nursing research, and nursing administration with regard to the primary nursing care modality.

I

THE EVOLUTION OF
NURSING CARE
MODALITIES

chapter 1

FACTORS INFLUENCING NURSING CARE MODALITIES

Nursing has searched for a delivery system that provides the best and most cost-effective care possible. To date, care delivery systems have been revised several times. Several factors affect both the development of a delivery system and its effectiveness in fulfilling needs of clients. Two of the most influential factors will be discussed in this chapter.

The first factor influencing nursing care delivery modes is the developmental stage of the profession. There are two aspects to professional development. The first aspect relates to the degree of attainment of professionalism; the second is the progression through successful attainment of developmental tasks, which parallel Erikson's human developmental tasks. These two areas of concern can provide clues about the ability of nursing to devise and enact a care system that is mature and professionally effective. If, for example, nursing has not completed one or more tasks of development, or if it does not meet one or more of the criteria for professionalism, does that limitation alter the potentiality for nursing to implement an effective delivery system? The answer, of course, is yes, since the degree to which nursing has successfully mastered developmental tasks and the degree to which it has attained professional maturity affects the extent to which it can respond to the needs of clients.

A second problem for nursing is the bureaucratic system of administration that is common in the environment in which nursing care systems have been devised. Nursing is practiced in hospitals, clinics, public health departments, industrial plants, schools, and other places. The dominant administrative patterns of these settings have been bureaucratic. Nursing, then, conformed to the administrative pattern of these agencies and failed to modify or depart from bureaucratic forms for delivery systems. The major nursing care patterns are highly reflective of these two problems: faulty professional development and bureaucratic managerial systems.

As nursing has matured, its practitioners have become more skilled and sophisticated in research, social systems dynamics, and organizational change strategies. Nurses have become more competent and confident in their ability to assay conditions and problems and to choose appropriate response patterns. Nursing accepts less passively the forces affecting nursing care delivery. Currently the response of nurses is to analyze change forces and to promote activities that will affect the change forces themselves. They have begun to formulate nursing care delivery systems that are more responsive to the needs of the client, the nurse, and the social system.

This chapter examines the two major forces affecting nursing care delivery modes and briefly describes the four most common nursing care delivery patterns.

PROFESSIONAL DEVELOPMENTAL STAGES AND NURSING CARE DELIVERY

Recent nursing history has been a progression or evolution through various phases of development. These phases of development are in two contiguous areas, and the ability of nursing to provide effective care depends on successful maturation in both areas. The first area is the evolution of the occupation toward professionalism, and the second is the successful attainment of various levels of tasks of development, paralleling Erikson's human developmental tasks.

The evolution of professionalism. Nursing's history has been one of growth toward professional maturity. There is a natural history of professions that each occupation enacts as it moves through time toward greater maturity. If at any point in its development an occupation fails to attain maturity, the occupation never develops to its fullest potential. It then remains occupational in nature, is absorbed by other professions, or disappears entirely.

Professionalism, as a title, is a prestige and status token; if this were the only role value of professionalization, then the question of whether nursing is a profession would not be important or germane to the question of nursing care administration. However, a useful purpose is served by looking carefully at the problem of professionalism. Since attainment of professional status marks maturity in the development of an occupational group and since maturity influences the effectiveness with which the group meets the needs of its clientele, then the criteria for measuring professional growth can provide important guidelines for measuring nursing care delivery modes.

An examination of the literature yields much data about nursing's status as a profession. Even articles dealing with other seemingly unrelated subjects provide material for measuring nursing to determine its professionalism. When one digests all the literature on professional criteria, a single pervasive and overriding concern exists: is the occupation able to be completely client-centered? Can it assess client needs and respond directly to those needs? In other words, the crux of the matter seems to be how well the occupation is organized to provide services that meet client needs. The ability of nursing to place the needs of patients first and to respond directly to those needs, rather than to the needs of medicine, government, or employing agencies, is the true test of maturity, that is, professionalism. Seen in this light, criteria for professionalism will help in determining the effectiveness of practice modes. The following list of five criteria for professionalism is a synthesis of the criteria devised by Flexner in 1915 and other later authors who have struggled with this same problem.[1]

1. Body of knowledge: Has a continually growing body of practice-oriented knowledge that is recognized by the client as necessary or useful to him
2. Collaboration: Collaborates with other service groups and individuals for the benefit of the patient, at the choice of the practitioner and/or the client
3. Colleagueship: Has strong peer colleagueship, demonstrated by (a) an organization that dictates licensing and practice laws designed to protect clients, promotes and improves the quality of practice, and provides a support system for its members; and (b) peer evaluation of its practitioners, designed to protect the safety of clients and provide care of the highest quality
4. Autonomy: Has autonomous practitioners who have direct lines of access to clients and who are responsible for their own practice decisions and accountable to clients, to peers, to the professional organization, and to the courts for their conduct
5. Ethics: Has a cohesive, clear, and well-articulated code of ethics voluntarily adhered to by members and designed to protect the client and his interests

According to these criteria, the area requiring most attention is that of autonomy. Autonomy for nursing will mean the ability to make decisions with the client without deference to others, unless the client or nurse chooses to collaborate on decision making. It will mean mutuality of access between client and practitioner without physician, hospital, principal, foreman, plant manager, supervisor, or director of nursing service acting as the gatekeeper of services. It will also mean direct responsibility for patient care and accountability to patients, to peer review boards, to the American Nurses Association, to the National League for Nursing, and to the courts for the type and quality of the care given. Autonomy will mean that nurses can and will provide nursing services to patients by responding to their needs and not to the needs of agencies or other professionals.

Developmental tasks for nursing. If the last hundred years of nursing history could be divided into growth and developmental stages, one would find striking parallels to Erikson's[2] tasks of human development. These tasks are trust, autonomy, industry and accomplishment, intimacy, identity, generativity, and integrity.

The development of a sense of *trust* requires an environment in which needs are consistently met. Nursing's early infancy was marked by a close paternal relationship with physicians and hospitals. Nurses gratefully accepted the protection, shelter, and teaching of physicians and institutions in the late nineteenth and early twentieth centuries. They were taught, nurtured, fed, clothed, and housed by hospitals employing them. This enabled nursing to develop a fairly strong sense of trust.

The establishment of *autonomy*, usually the second task of development, was all but omitted from the growth pattern. Small efforts to establish autonomy were made in the 1930s when public health nursing came into existence. Autonomy, however, was never accepted as a legitimate characteristic of nursing, and therefore this task of development was not attained.

The sense of *industry and accomplishment,* a stage reached by engaging in real, worthwhile, socially useful tasks that can be completed with pride, came to nursing in the 1920s and 1930s. At that time nursing began to move into universities; it began to study the social health care needs in the country and to try to respond to them. The sense of industry and accomplishment was closely tied to the development of a sense of *identity.* The growing profession attempted to clarify what it was, its role in the world, its position in the health care spectrum, and where and to what groups it belonged. The need to complete these two tasks of development spawned studies of nursing, nursing education, and nursing activities. Everything was studied, from education and service deficiencies to procedures and functions. These studies served to develop both the sense of industry and accomplishment and the sense of identity. One consequence of the studies was that the parameters of nursing gradually began to emerge, and the functional differences and likenesses between nursing and other health disciplines began to be delineated.

The next task of development to be attempted was the sense of *intimacy.* In this stage the developing profession established warm, close bonds with others. Feeling a need for these relationships, nursing developed close ties with sociologists, psychologists, physiologists, chemists, and biologists. Nursing degrees were limited to the master's level, and nurses desiring further education chose anthropology, sociology, education, psychology, and the biological sciences. This marriage of disciplines had good consequences. It produced people skilled in scientific methods and brought sociological and anthropological research methods to nursing problems and scientific training to nursing practitioners, enabling them to bring a scientific approach to the solving of nursing care problems. It was primarily responsible for the growth of the body of knowledge in nursing and the attainment of a sense of identity. It was the impetus behind the change in focus in nursing education from content memorization to the process of problem solving. This bond with other groups enabled nursing to experience the power of close professional ties with allied groups and colleagues in those groups. Friends of nursing from other disciplines contributed immeasurably to nursing.

Nursing's age of *generativity,* which developed simultaneously with the sense of intimacy and identity, is illustrated in the entry of nursing ancillary workers into the care giving scene. Nursing shortages in World War II provided the impetus for the explosion of ancillary workers. Even had there been no war and no resultant acute shortage of personnel, ancillary workers would probably have evolved, for health care demands were growing, since people of every social strata began to seek quality health care on an equal footing with the rich or privileged. Demands outstripped supply, and nursing was caught short. The evolution might have been slower and the ancillary workers fewer in number without the war, but because the population was increasing and health care demands expanding beyond the ability of nursing to respond, the technician was born.

Unfortunately there was no planned specific effort to study the demands of society or to gauge the needs of consumers and employers of nursing service or any organized systematic emergence of roles; rather, there was a simple spinning off of some of the more technical tasks for economy of time and money. It was an occupational "happening." Operating room technicians, psychiatric technicians, corpsmen, aides, and vocational nurses came into being. Now almost every technical task in the health care and nursing fields has its technicians. Nursing still acts as parent to some of these fields; it is the nurse who teaches the vocational nurse, the nurse who teaches aides, the nurse who teaches operating room technicians, and the nurse who teaches many other technical workers. There will come a time when, like children, these groups come of age and move into their own independence and territory.

However, the problem of nursing autonomy still remains. Since nursing did not complete the growth and development task of autonomy at the proper stage, and autonomy is a necessary feature of professionalism, that task must still be attained, or maturity can never be achieved. Professionally, *the lack of autonomy is the key to nursing's arrested development.* Any nursing practice system that lacks that key ingredient will not provide adequate services to consumers or fulfill the needs of the nurses themselves. When autonomy is attained, nursing can achieve maturity—a healthy, integrated personality and a system of care that accepts life, limitations, and potential, works in its time period, and totally utilizes its population of practitioners.

Despite the fact that the sequence of development for autonomy is out of order, nursing is currently growing in autonomy. Trends in the delivery of nursing care are clear expressions of this growth. All new modes of nursing care delivery are toward increased autonomy and the increased assumption of direct responsibility and authority for assessing, diagnosing, and solving nursing problems and prescribing nursing actions. Nurses are getting the requisite preparation, taking the risks, separating from hospitals and traditional agencies, and setting up business as independent providers of direct care to patients. Nurses in every setting are demanding direct access to patients and demanding that patients have direct access to them.

The expanded role of the nurse is to be treated not as a physician's assistant but as the patient's assistant. *Colleagueship* with other health-related disciplines is the key, and *autonomy* is its major characteristic. Both colleagueship and autonomy are essential ingredients for professionalism.

BUREAUCRACY AND NURSING CARE DELIVERY

Nursing has been influenced not only by its own growth and development periodicity but by its context. Nursing in the United States arose in a period of industrialization and mass production. It was born and weaned in a milieu of bureaucracies and had to pass through all the stages of development in bureaucracies. Therefore it is a product of and reflects the bureaucratic system of management that characterizes the era. Bureaurcracy is a mark of the armed forces, government, business, most churches, and health agencies alike. Each of these institutions adopted bureaucratic forms from early military patterns. It seems natural that nursing, an integral part of a society so permeated with bureaucratic managerial systems, should have these same traits. Bureaucracies have four basic characteristics: (1) hierarchical line authority, (2) specific divisions of labor, (3) authority delegated with responsibility, and (4) pyramidal supervisory structure. Most current nursing care delivery modes demonstrate these same elements.

Hierarchical line of authority. This managerial system has been fraught with problems for the nursing profession. Here, ultimate responsibility for all decisions and actions remains with the person at the head of the line. The "buck" of decision making and blame can be passed up and down the line until the decision timing is off; thus crises develop, or decisions are made by default.

Another problem is that decisions can be made at the "top" by people in positions of authority to be carried out by the people at the "bottom." This decision-making shuttle system is a slow response pattern. The decision "cop out" is common because it is possible to remove decision making from the person to whom the work has been delegated. Unfortunately for nursing, especially in formalized health agencies, the line authority communication pattern is highly confused. The nurse is employed by the agency and subject to its line of authority. Specifically, the chain of responsibility flows from administrator to nursing director to supervisor to head nurse to staff nurse. The care giver is paid by this formal organizational structure and must respond to its organizational format. By tradition and sometimes by legal dictates the nurse is directly responsible to the physician who acts as controller of health care for patients and who delegates, by "orders," specific responsibilities to nurses. Nurses who do not respond to this authority are subject to pressure from physicians and other nurses, as well as legal action by the courts. Conflicts between hospital policy and physicians' "orders" often catch the nurse in a decision bind. Professionally the nurse is responsible to the patient, and ethically the line of authority stops with that relationship.

When private duty nurses are employed directly by the client, it is usually a direct result of physicians' orders, and payment is made frequently by an insurance company. This fourth party, the insurance company, further muddies the water. Since the fee comes from the insurance company, should the company be considered the nurse's employer, or is the nurse employed by the client to whom the services are rendered? Unfortunately, because of blurred and ill-defined bureaucratic policy, the average staff nurse has three "bosses"—the employing agency, the physician, and the patient. The average private duty nurse also has three bosses—the insurance company, the physician, and the patient.

Specific divisions of labor. Bureaucratic divisions of labor are usually by territory. These can be divided by function or by geography. The automobile assembly line is an example of the territoriality of function concept carried to an extreme. Hospitals have been patterned on this system with personnel who specialize in dietetics, x-ray, housekeeping, etc. Division of labor by function became a mark of the health care bureaucracy. Procedure manuals are perhaps one of the most distinct earmarks of the division-of-labor characteristic. Such manuals describe every task in detail, and explicit directions are given for performing each task so that minions down the hierarchical scale need not exercise any judgement; all they have to do is follow the procedure as described. Nurses have long thought they invented the procedure manual; they did not. They simply conformed to the methods of the other bureaucracies. Every bureaucracy has its own procedure manual.

Another way to divide labor has been by geography. Typical of the territoriality by geography concept is the system used by salesmen. State maps divided by colored lines marking specific jurisdictions ensure that a salesman does not intrude into another's territory. Hospitals have also used this approach, especially with the head nurse and supervisory staff. Basic responsibility for a geographical area has been as respected in nursing as it is among sales forces. Supervisors are given responsibility for certain nursing stations or "floors." Every kind of nursing problem in that territory is the responsibility of the supervisor. Whether the supervisor has any expertise in specific kinds of problems does not matter. The patients and nurses within the territorial boundaries of a supervisor are the supervisor's responsibility. Not until recently has supervision been seen as a method for providing consultation that can overlap both function and geography.

In divisions of labor both by geography and function, delegation of a territory includes delegation of authority to perform tasks germane to the specific territory. The problems that have resulted are organically connected to the paradox between the holistic nature of man and the functional division of responses to man's needs. For example, the director of in-service education is responsible for staff development; the supervisor is responsible for supervising staff to produce quality care; the in-service director promises not to supervise, and the supervisor promises not to teach. Does no one think of the staff nurse who, to grow, needs a resource person, not a policeman? That resource person cannot separate consultation, validation, and generation of alternatives from teaching and still be effective.

Authority delegated with responsibility. Typically bureaucratic systems have delegated the authority to act and to make decisions as they delegated the responsibilities for particular functions or territories. It is at all times, however, a delegated responsibility with an "out." The final (sometimes referred to in the literature as "ultimate") responsibility can move up the line of organization. Generally, however, a person delegated to a function or a geography is provided with both the authority to make decisions and the authority to carry out measures necessary to the successful accomplishment of the task.

The responsibility and authority are related only to the employee's job description, which is tied to such remarkable phenomena as status, tenure, rank, and place in the corporate structure. In other words, the authority and responsibilities delegated may be totally unrelated to capability. Thus the natural well of knowledge and skill from which true authority springs is not necessarily the fountain from which authority delegated by the bureaucracy flows. This can and does lead to conflicts between those with delegated power and those with natural power of knowledge, skill, and leadership ability. Decisions are sometimes made in response to other than direct job needs. They are, for example, made to conform to the corporate pattern, policies, and what looks good for the decision maker and the company. They are not always made on the lines of the most appropriate alternative for the situation.

Policy manuals mark this bureaucratic characteristic. Like procedure manuals, policy manuals are part of every bureaucratic system. The limited autonomy discussed previously is further compromised by "policing by policy." Guidelines for making decisions are established, and all contingencies are provided for so that true freedom to respond to a problem with a solution tailored to a specific case is all but removed from the decision maker. Thus bureaucracies are characterized by delegating authority with responsibility to people who can pass decisions along to higher echelons if the policy manual is not clear about the guidelines.

Pyramidal supervisory structure. The biblical King David set captains over tens, captains over hundreds, and captains over thousands. Bureaucratic supervisory structures seem to have altered little since the campaigns of Saul and David. This pattern of "overseer," in which one supervisor oversees the work of several workers, permeates almost all work settings. The name may be foreman, pusher, supervisor, boss, or captain, but the pattern remains the same. The typical pyramid of authority and overseeing has several workers under one supervisor, several supervisors under one higher supervisor, several higher supervisors under one assistant to the chief, and several assistants to the chief under the chief. The system survives because it is impossible for one director of nursing to communicate directly with 100 to 200 nurses. The communication problems would become astronomical. Therefore the pyramid system has achieved at least one goal—providing channels of communication for people along the "chain of command." The system has a disease, however, the disease of "creeping top weight." Creeping top weight infects the system because the more supervisors there are, the more supervisors are needed to supervise the supervisors. Fig. 1-1 illustrates this point.

Creeping top weight is a costly disease both in personnel numbers and salaries. The more supervisors there are (usually at higher salaries), the fewer people there are giving direct patient care. No one has yet established a magic ratio of supervisors to nurses or to patients. Different numbers work differently in different settings. An optimal number will probably never be established because problems, clients, geography, and the type of nursing care delivery system varies widely from setting to setting.

The bureaucratic mark of such pyramiding is the job description. Job descriptions are a symptom of all bureaucracies, since with so many people in the pyramid, the overlap and blurring of territory and functions become a problem.

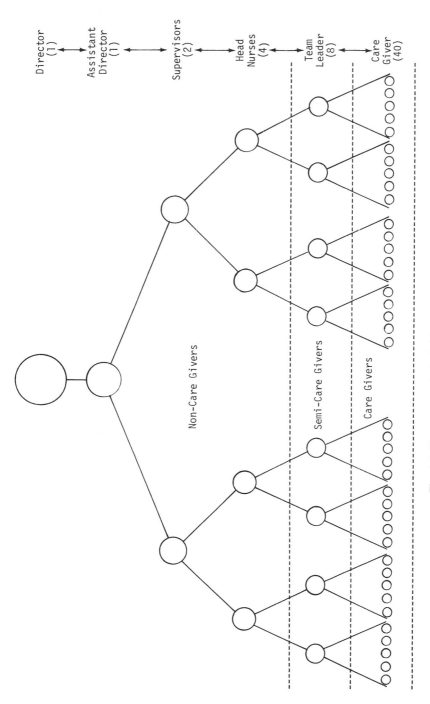

Director
(1)

Assistant
Director
(1)

Supervisors
(2)

Head
Nurses
(4)

Team
Leader
(8)

Care
Giver
(40)

Non-Care Givers

Semi-Care Givers

Care Givers

Fig. 1-1. Team pyramid of administrators and care givers.

Careful definition of job responsibility therefore is necessary. The job description tells the employee who he is, to whom he reports, what functions he performs, and the parameters of his responsibilities.

Job descriptions for nurses at all levels must be changed if nursing care delivery modes are to change. Furthermore, reeducation of nurses in all positions must occur. Care givers must be taught how to make nursing care decisions, using problem-solving strategies that enable them to make the best possible decision for the patient at that time. Some of the pyramid structure must disappear. Many of those in the higher echelons, especially team leaders, can become care givers themselves; some, notably the supervisors, can become specialty area experts; some can become experts in problem solving. Therefore care givers can have help when they wish it in identifying problems, gathering and sorting data, generating alternatives, and choosing and implementing alternatives. The traditional roles of the hierarchical decision maker will change.

NURSING CARE DELIVERY MODES

Nursing care delivery modes have reflected the lack of professionalism, the stage of development in nursing wherein the system became prominent, and the bureaucratic context of nursing administration.

Historically there have been and still are many organizational patterns for the delivery of nursing care. Only four of these have been commonly used to an extent worthy of comment: (1) the case modality, (2) the functional modality, (3) the team modality, and (4) the primary nursing care modality.

Case modality. The case method was the earliest form of nursing care, dating back to the years when the sense of trust was being developed. This method enabled the nurse to plan and administer care to the patient on a one-to-one basis. The case method has persisted, especially in schools of nursing where it has been used as the vehicle for teaching "idealized" patient care to students. It is also used in acute care settings, especially in intensive care units. It has persisted in some hosptials where other forms of care have never been allowed to intrude.

As just indicated, one method does not necessarily disappear as other methods emerge. Like human developmental phases, the care delivery methods persist, overlap, and continue in both mixed and pure forms in nursing agencies.

Functional modality. Functional nursing care arose during the time when nursing was developing a sense of industry, accomplishment, and identity. Studies in the 1920s, 1930s, and early 1940s gave rise to functional divisions of labor that almost depersonalized nursing. If Henry Ford could turn out automobiles on an assembly line using a functional approach, why could nursing not be made more efficient by adopting the same approach? Time and motion studies thrived, and efficiency was viewed apart from the context of patient needs. Divsion of labor was determined by technical aspects of the job to be done. For example, one nurse administered medications, one gave treatments, one changed water pitchers, another served meal trays, another changed beds, and others bathed patients.

The functional method of delivering nursing care was a direct outgrowth of the division of labor by task. The bureaucratic system of mass production, which involves attention to quantity, de-emphasis on quality, and the one man for one task specialization idea, was adopted by nursing. The outcome was the ability to take the technical functions of nursing and sort them into levels of complexity. The aide was given the simplest tasks that took little training; the vocational nurse was given the next level of function, those tasks requiring more training but that were not too complex; the registered nurse was given the most complex functions. Each person responded to his function, and little attention was provided to the patient who in the course of a day had to deal with four or five care givers, of whom none had particular responsibility for him as a unique whole person. His humanism was mechanized; his organismic whole was fractured into parts; his basic physiological and technical needs were reduced to a checklist on paper. Thus he became the automated patient. One such patient was heard to quip: "In and out for an appendectomy in three days and never touched by human hands."

Team modality. During the developmental stage of generativity, team nursing was born. World War II receded, leaving behind a host of health care workers trained in a variety of technical skills on a wide range of levels. Hospitals had absorbed droves of these workers to help ease the acute nursing shortages of the war years. In essence, they found technicians, vocational nurses, and aides a cheap source of labor. The quality of nursing care suffered from inadequate preparation for the nursing care given. There were not enough nurses to do the job and not enough supervisors and head nurses to provide adequate supervision to poorly trained personnel. Team nursing seemed an answer to a profession in a care delivery crisis. Several nurses, orderlies, aides, and vocational nurses were put under the supervision of one nurse, the team leader, to provide care to a group of patients. Ideally the team leader was the best prepared person and was expected to facilitate the team in formulating and carrying out nursing care plans for every patient assigned to the team. Realistically, however, the demands of the job were far too great for one individual to fulfill. The team leader had to know not only the diagnosis, medications, orders, and tests on each patient but also the family problems and the social and ethnic background. She had to compile a nursing history and help the team formulate a nursing care plan for each patient. Further duties included supervision of the activities of others to ensure that the plan was enacted. On top of these duties, the nurse also had to give and receive reports, plan relief for team members (lunch and coffee breaks), hold nursing care planning conferences, and, in some cases, give medications, treatments, and/or other care to patients. In many agencies the team leader was also the person primarily responsible for in-service education. It is not surprising that few nursing care plans were written or that those written were superficial and general, sometimes merely a repetition of the physician's orders. The team leader had little time to see that those written plans could be adequately carried out.

The pyramidal supervisory structure is the perfect pattern for team nursing, for one nurse leader guides and supervises the work of several care givers. Most team leaders consider themselves nursing care givers, but time actually spent in the administering of care to patients is minimal. This is not surprising in view of the span of duties just listed. It would take a "supernurse" complete with telephone booth for changing from an ordinary ward clerk to the uniform of "supernurse" to perform the many functions required during the normal day of a team leader. Actual time spent with patients is secondary to the supervisory functions of the team leader.

Primary nursing modality. Primary nursing care belongs to the developmental stage of maturity. Through primary nursing the potentials of nursing care are beginning to be realized. Limitations and strengths are viewed realistically, with people and practitioners being a part of the total potential personality of nursing. The missing element in the development of professional autonomy is being discovered. Primary nursing, like case method care, assigns one nurse to each patient. Whereas the case method nurse may be responsible for her shift only, the primary nurse is responsible for the patient twenty-four hours a day for the duration of the care need or length of hospitalization. The primary care nurse assesses the patient's nursing care needs, collaborates with the patient and other health personnel, and formulates a plan of care that the nurse is responsible for carrying out around the clock every day. The primary nurse may delegate to a secondary nurse the responsibility for executing the care plan on other shifts, but delegation is accomplished by means of nursing care plans, notes, recordings, etc., and never proceeds through a supervisorial third person. Thus the primary care nurse is a "triple A" nurse, having three basic characteristics: *A*utonomy, *A*uthority, and *A*ccountability.

The primary nurse has *autonomy* in that care is based on a nursing care plan worked out between the primary nurse and the patient. Collaboration with other health care givers, such as the physician, dietician, physical therapist, occupational therapist, and other relevant persons, is close and continuing. But the activity is collaborative, not subordinative, and is performed in a colleague relationship. The primary nurse has complete control of the care giving at all times. Other nurses become resources to the primary nurse, and problem solving, validating, sharing of expertise, and other collaborative practices mark intraprofessional relationships. Head nurses and supervisors become nursing care consultants, not people-watching policemen and administrative errand boys. Direct client-nurse access has not yet been achieved but is possible if nurses persist.

The primary nurse has *authority* in that responsibility for care involves the totality of that care, that is, the comprehensive nursing care plan and its implementation on a twenty-four-hour basis for as long as care is needed. The primary nurse is responsible to the patient for the quality of care, for meeting care agreements, and for continuity of care, whether or not the primary nurse is on duty. The primary care nurse assumes this responsibility as consistent with her role. There is no pyramiding of hierarchical decision makers. Decisions are participatory, involving patients and care givers most directly concerned with the care.

The primary nurse makes and is *accountable* for all decisions regarding patients in her care. Collaborating with others is a matter of choice by the nurse and does not relieve the nurse of the responsibility. The proverbial "buck" cannot be passed; it rests with the nurse providing care. Every decision has its consequences and every nursing act its payoff. In other systems the dispersion of authority and lack of autonomy have relieved nurses of the opportunity to be accountable for their own behaviors. Often the payoff or the consequences of decisions were never known to the decision makers. The rewards or punishments of a sequel to a care plan or a decision may have been known only to the nurse on a given shift or another service. This left nurses with little sense of reinforcement and with few reliable feedback loops. Care could not improve systematically because the essential device—feedback—was missing or erratic.

Accountability means standing behind decisions and actions. When one nurse is responsible, consequences are funneled back, and the payoff, good or bad, rests with the primary nurse.

SUMMARY AND IMPLICATIONS

Hierarchical line authority has permeated nursing culture for most of its existence, making it easy for nurses to abort the development of autonomy. The nurse could relinquish all responsibility simply by following physicians' orders or supervisors' dictates. Autonomy is inseparable from the assumption of responsibility and accountability for one's own acts, which are both marks of professionalism. Therefore, when nurses allowed others to take the responsibility, they surrendered their autonomy. When functional and team nursing became common delivery modes, nurses could not only pass decision-making responsibility to physicians and administrators, they could pass it to team leaders. The game, "You make the decisions, I'll do the griping," became popular because care givers could, according to both tradition and policy, allow others to make decisions concerning the care of their patients. Then, when things did not go well, the care giver could persecute the person in higher authority for making a wrong decision.

Any nursing care delivery system that insists on care givers' assuming the responsibility for decisions regarding the plan of care and implementation of that plan for their patients must change the hierarchical line of authority.

Nursing's conformity to bureaucracy manifests the characteristics of line authority, task-oriented care, responsibility delegated with function, and pyramidal supervisory structure. This bureaucratic nurse can make whatever decisions are necessary, as long as they do not intrude on the territory (geographical or functional) of other personnel and as long as they come within the job description of his/her position. Decisions can be made by the nurse insofar as there are guidelines for those decisions in the policy manual, insofar as there are directions for carrying out these decisions in the procedures manual, and insofar as the nurse has the approval of his or her supervisor. On this basis alone, nursing is, and has been for decades, ripe for change to a better care delivery system. However, the bureaucratic characteristics are characteristics that provide stability to a system. It is not a system that is geared to rapid change, flexibility, innovation, experimentation, and different responses to problems. The whole point of bureaucracy is to provide a stable, surviving mechanism. The paradox is that the very stability that helps the system survive for a time chokes it in time. It is not strange, however, that nursing adopted two systems of care that are reflections of the context in which nursing takes place. Born in a society that is mass producing, housed in agencies that are bureaucratic, and lacking the developmental task of autonomy, nursing devised two delivery systems that were direct outgrowths of these characteristics: functional and team nursing.

REFERENCES

1. These criteria represent a synthesis of ideas from the following:
    Flexner, Abraham: Is social work a profession? Proceedings of the National Conference of Charities and Correction, 1915, pp. 578-581.
    Baldridge, J. Victor: Professionalism, a lecture given at Stanford University, Palo Alto, Calif., Oct. 23, 1969.
    Goode, William J.: The theoretical limits of professionalization. In Etzioni, Amitai, editor: The semi-professions and their organization, New York, 1969, The Free Press, pp. 266-313.
    Norris, Catherine M.: Direct access to the patient, American Journal of Nursing 70:1006-1010, 1970.
2. Erikson, E. H.: Childhood and society, ed. 2, New York, 1950, W. W. Norton & Co., Inc., pp. 247-273.

SUGGESTED READINGS

Angrist, Shirley: Nursing care: the dream and the reality. In Lewis, Edith P.: Changing patterns of nursing practice: new needs, new roles, New York, 1971, The American Journal of Nursing Co., pp. 142-149.
Davis, Fred., editor: The nursing profession, New York, 1966, John Wiley & Sons, Inc.
Dilworth, Ava S.: Goals for nursing. In Dryden, M. Virginia, editor: Nursing trends, Dubuque, 1968, William C. Brown Co., pp. 41-53.
Douglas, Laura Mae, and Bevis, Em Olivia: Nursing leadership in action, St. Louis, 1974, The C. V. Mosby Co.
Edelstein, Ruth: Automation: its effect on the nurse. In Lewis, Edith P.: Changing patterns of nursing practice: new needs, new roles, New York, 1971, The American Journal of Nursing Co., pp. 269-277.
Fagin, Claire M., and Goodwin, Beatrice: Baccalaureate preparation for primary care, Nursing Outlook 20:240-244, April, 1972.
Fritz, Edna: Baccalaureate nursing education: what is its job? In Dryden, M. Virginia, editor: Nursing trends, Dubuque, 1968, William C. Brown Co., pp. 199-207.
Glasser, Melvin A.: Consumer expectations of health services. In Corey, Lawrence, Saltman, Steven E., and Epstein, Michael F., editors: Medicine in a changing society, St. Louis, 1923, The C. V. Mosby Co., pp. 29-38.
Kramer, Marlene: The new graduate speaks again, American Journal of Nursing 69:1903-1907, 1969.
Lenninger, M. M., Little, D. E., and Carnevalie, Doris: Primex, American Journal of Nursing 72:1274-1277, 1972.
Logsdon, Audrey: Why primary nursing? Nursing Clinics of North America 8:283-291, 1973.
Manallen, Helen K.: The changing role of the nurse, In Lewis, Edith P.: Changing patterns

of nursing practice: new needs, new roles, New York, 1971, The American Journal of Nursing Co., pp. 93-99.

Manthey, Marie, Ciske, Karen, Robertson, Patricia, and Harris, Isabel: Primary nursing: a return to the concept of "my nurse" and "my patient," Nursing Forum **9:**65-83, 1970.

Marram, Gwen D.: Innovation on Four Tower West: what happened? American Journal of Nursing **73:**814-816, 1973.

Marram, Gwen D.: Patients' evaluation of their care—importance to the nurse, Nursing Outlook **21:**322-325, May, 1973.

Mumford, Lewis: Automation and society. In Bryant, Clifton D., editor: Social problems today: dilemmas and discussions, New York, 1971, J. B. Lippincott Co., pp. 54-56.

Murray, B. Louise: A case for independent group nursing practice, Nursing Outlook **20:**60-63, Jan., 1972.

Strauss, Anselm: The structure and ideology of American nursing: an interpretation. In Davis, Fred, editor: The nursing profession: five sociological essays, New York, 1966, John Wiley & Sons. Inc., pp. 60-108.

U. S. Department of Health, Education and Welfare: Extending the scope of nursing practice, Nursing Outlook **20:**46-52, Jan., 1972.

Waters, Verle Hambleton: Distinctions are necessary. In Dryden, M. Virginia, editor: Nursing trends, Dubuque, 1968, William C. Brown Co., pp. 219-222.

Wolford, Helen: The nurse of the future. In Lewis, Edith P.: Changing patterns of nursing practice: new needs, new roles, New York, 1971, The American Journal of Nursing Co., pp. 100-104.

chapter 2

THE SOCIAL CONTEXT OF NURSING AND CRITERIA FOR AN OPTIMUM NURSING CARE SYSTEM

Chapter 1 stressed the role of autonomy, its absence, and the consequential lack of success of nursing care delivery systems. The deficient characteristic autonomy cannot be considered apart from the social context that inhibits its flourishing. When considered as a part of the total picture of the role of women in Western civilization and in light of the complete control of client access held by medicine, the problem of autonomy gains perspective and becomes more real. Autonomy is the next goal to be achieved by nursing, and, before marked improvement in nursing care can be attained, a means of increasing nursing's autonomy must be found.

Accessibility to clients was also highlighted as a central problem. Accessibility lines between client and nurse will ensure that autonomy can be practiced and that nurses will have authority to provide care that is quality controlled by their own peers. Accessibility to date has been barred by the traditional powers given to medicine by custom and law.

The control of patient accessibility is only one result of medicine's domination in the health care field. The second problem arising from that ideology is the dualistic approach to man, in which he is considered by age, physiological system, diagnosis, or stage of illness instead of as an organismic whole. Most health care groups have followed the lead of medicine and have treated patients in parts and pieces.

These are problems that inhibit the creation of satisfactory nursing care systems but need not be allowed to block their evolution. This evolution cannot be left to chance, and to ensure that nursing care systems are generated that do meet needs of clients, a definitive set of criteria must be devised. Criteria for a system must be derived from the characteristics of the social context in which the system is to function. With a list of criteria, the care delivery system can be measured to determine areas that need continuing alteration to be optimally effective.

This chapter contains a discussion of the traditional role of women in American life and the resulting influence on nursing. It presents a brief discussion of some problems that arise in nursing because of the dominance of physicians as the guard to health care access. Finally, it presents a suggested list of criteria by which to measure a nursing care delivery system to determine its effectiveness in meeting needs of clients. The summary includes an analysis of the implications for nursing in the implementation of such a care system.

MALE-DOMINATED SOCIETY

The title by which the profession is addressed is a feminine gender title: *nurse*. Nurse usually refers to a female who takes care of children or feeds them at the breast. The title evolved to mean those who cared for children and the sick. However, the name, true to its origin, communicates female servant images. Men in nursing have long objected to the title, and some women have joined their ranks; however, no one has succeeded in renaming the group. Many problems that have consistently recurred in nursing through the years are directly attributable to the male-female role definition within the society of Western civilization. This clearly is not a problem that nursing can attribute to men or to society in general. Everyone has participated in making the male domination in society successful, and nursing has been an active player in role taking. Men are not more culpable in the social role system problem than are women. Role-connected injustices for men are pervasive in society, just as they are for women. However, it is the influence of this problem on nursing and therefore on the female inequities that is germane here.

It takes three to make a role: the player, the complementary role, and the audience. Each person in society plays all three roles at various times. Each role requires the player to know the complementary role and further requires that the complementary role be enacted. Thus the nurse must know the physician role (the nurses' complementary role) if the nurse is to enact her role properly. The converse is true also; the physician must know the nurse role, for unless the complementary role of nurse is properly enacted, the role of the male (dominating) physician cannot be enacted. The implications are that unless the nurse complements the male-dominating role by allowing herself to be the foil for domination, then the male dominating role cannot be enacted. Thus the great trick society plays on women is that they become participants in their own devaluation.

The male-female role definition in Western society has probably influenced the lack of autonomy in nursing more than any other single factor. Autonomy is difficult for women to attain because of the cultural and social context of their lives. Historically women were not allowed independence. Guardianship was transferred from father or other male designee to husband on marriage, and the woman was never allowed to control her own finances. The traditional marriage ceremony to this day asks: "Who gives this woman to be wed to this man?" This implies that the father, uncle, or brother has the right to "give" the female member of the family to the keeping of another male and thereby transfer responsibility to him. Although the legal restraints have largely disappeared, some states still have marriage laws that require married women to conduct certain of their business activities jointly with their husbands. This tradition persists in attitude, if not in practice, influencing all male-female relationships, especially business and professional ones. The idealized female role in our society is characterized by the image of a compassionate, soft, sweet, devoted, dependent, and accepting weaker human. The successful professional woman, by contrast, is commonly presumed (by other women as well as men) to have avoided these virtues in favor of the aggressive, hard, independent, castrating, and unsympathetic nonfeminine characteristics. She has become, in short, the antithesis of "what a woman should be." Through the preset, culturally conditioned eyes of most people, this perception is palpably dehumanizing, having little or nothing to do with the personal characteristics of the individual woman. Expectably, since no woman wishes to be viewed as nonfeminine, the messages are transmitted by way of the old cultural channels: "Do not assert yourself!" and "Do not be independent or autonomous!" It is anomalous that social presets allow men to be aggressive and independent, yet loving, compassionate, and supportive, and women who are aggressive and independent cannot be perceived as capable of possessing other humanistic characteristics.

Women are perhaps more punitive to each other than are men. Women who successfully break the social role set represent to other women an enviable state and thus are a threat; this envy gives rise to the following ambivalence: admiration on the one hand and jealousy on the other. The constant sense of failure to break out of the mold and the desire, yet fear of so doing, cause mixed feelings that are difficult to deal with constructively. Therefore the successful woman in a predominantly female profession such as nursing receives many mixed messages from her colleagues, ranging from rage and hate to admiration and affection. The risk of professional success therefore is high. As social consciousness develops, discussions of the problem have become easier, and relationship maintenance and mutual support systems have become a deliberate and legitimate endeavor.

Nevertheless, it is easy to see that with such social pressures, women have been reluctant to establish autonomy. Autonomy would necessitate fighting against the social context, giving up for a while the "ideal woman" image, and becoming and acting independent and responsible. Nurses, like women in general, are in the process of trying their wings of independence by taking another look at the developmental task of autonomy.

This whole role preset of society and its mechanisms for maintaining the stability of these roles has been a major factor in several other problems in nursing. Probably the easiest to pinpoint is professional sabotage, that is, insidious destruction of the profession. Professional sabotage occurs because of several socially indoctrinated attitudes in women.

Life expectations. Most women who choose nursing as a career are, like other young women, expecting to be active in that career only temporarily. Since it is often believed that the woman's primary goal is to marry, have children, and not work outside the home while the children are growing up, there is little enduring lifetime commitment to nursing. It is a temporary expedient solution to education and employment. Nursing does, as a side effect, stand a woman in good stead for preparing her for wifehood and motherhood. This lack of commitment to life-time employment leads to tolerance of undesirable working conditions within the profession. A more realistic look at the twenty-year working career of the average woman would indicate to most nurses that working conditions are not temporary and are worthy of the time and energy necessary to make changes for the better.

Acceptance of the myth of womens' salaries as supplements to family income. Salaries have only recently begun to come into the acceptable range and still are not at a good life maintenance level in many parts of the country. Because the nurse's view was short-range, her salary was seen as supplementary to her husband's and temporary or intermittent in nature. Retirement policies, social security, insurance, vacation, and leave allotments along with other fringe benefits that are normal parts of employment in large industries are absent or minimal for nurses. These conditions have been tolerated by nurses for many reasons. Primarily because of socially preset life expectations, nurses have viewed working in their profession as a temporary and undesirable condition and there-fore have not actively participated in attempts to alter conditions.

Career as a form of "fail-safe" life insurance. The life insurance phenomenon has been a benefit to women in the fulfillment of their wife-mother roles and a liability to professional standards. Women have chosen nursing for many reasons. One reason has been, "I can always nurse," meaning that when all else fails, when children grow up and no longer need mothering, if the breadwinner dies or becomes unable to support the family fully, or if times grow difficult, the nurse can, after years of absence, take up nursing again. This alone has damaged the profession; women long absent from practice lose their skills and forget content. Content changes so rapidly that an absence of two years makes much phar-macological and technological knowledge obsolete. As a consequence, nursing is shortchanged by the women who use it as insurance. As a "fail-safe" mecha-nism, it has not been a priority commitment and has not received the energy, time, effort, and active participation necessary for improvement of conditions, improvement of standards, improvement in patient care, and increase of practical knowledge. It has been used badly; much has been taken from nursing by this behavior, and little has been contributed. Actually the housewife-mother could, if willing to avail herself of the opportunity, contribute much to nursing during those childbearing, childrearing years. She could give nursing the same priority she gives a charity, volunteer work, or her bridge club. She could work with professional standards committees, special interest groups, research groups, etc., and make a substantial contribution to nursing. Insofar as nursing is viewed as an insurance policy and not as a major interest and commitment item, it is filed in the safety deposit box with the other insurance policies and locked there until needed.

Nursing's low-priority status. Often the working mother gives nursing the third priority to husband and children. If the children are sick, it is mother who stays at home with them. Few men stay away from work to take care of the sick child. If the husband is ill, the wife stays away from work and takes care of him. If the husband is transferred to another city by his firm, the wife resigns and moves with him. Few men are asked by their wives to move to a city where they can continue as nurses in a health care system that has widespread branches. Few couples when choosing a place to live do so with the career of the wife in mind. However, many more couples are looking for locations where both wife and husband are equally well situated with regard to desirable career placements. This low-priority status, which is deemed right and acceptable by society, accepted and approved by women, and thereby perpetuated with their consent, has deprived nursing and other women's professions of commitment and continuity.

Woman's role, woman's work, woman's place. The "woman's role, woman's work, woman's place" syndrome is an attitude of both women and men that has produced additional problems for nursing. The attitude of "woman's work" made nursing readily accept and continue to perpetuate housekeeping chores as part of nursing responsibility. Since housekeeping, like nursing, was accepted as woman's work, it was unquestioningly incorporated into nursing duties. Even though most agencies have separate departments that are assigned housekeeping chores and responsibilities, any survey of the average acute care hospital will show the nurse still performing many housekeeping chores. Changing beds for ambulatory patients, cleaning the bedside table, replenishing supplies, straightening and dusting the room when the hygienic care is completed, and even taking care of flower arrangements are all housekeeping chores.

The woman's role training in the life social structure has conditioned men and women to relate to each other in stereotyped patterns. The traditional male-female roles are seductive, father-daughter, or mother-father-child relationships. Any observer on a typical acute care nursing unit will see evidence of these role options.

The father-mother-child relationship is played out in many nurse-physician-patient situations. The patient becomes the child, the nurse the mother, and the physician the father. The physician plays the part of major decision maker, sustainer, and provider. The nurse is the nurturer, counselor, and manipulator of the physician on behalf of the patient. The patient becomes the child whose civil rights are removed and for whom all decisions are made. Fortunately the patient does not want to be treated like a child and is therefore demanding a participatory role; the nurse does not want to play mother and is demanding a participatory role; and many physicians are now resisting the father image and seek collaboration with others.

The nurse manipulates the physician and the physician manipulates the nurse by means of the seductive behaviors common in the dominant white middle-class society. Physicians call the nurse "honey." They flirt with her, tell her how pretty she looks, and are thoughtful on holidays, bringing candy for special occasions like Christmas. The nurse reciprocates and often initiates the seductive behavior.

The patronizing father-daughter relationship, is perhaps even more common than seduction. This is the "father knows all, sees all, cares about everything, and will take care of everything" attitude. The "putdown" is not intentional because this relationship is basically a kind one, full of good feelings for both players. The "putdown" inherent in patronization is cushioned in layers of kindness. Therein lies its insidious malignancy. No bonds are so difficult to break as those of kindness. It is the child smothered with love who finds it most difficult to leave home, not the child who is treated with some degree of peerage or benign neglect. The other problem of patronization is the high cost nursing pays for the comfortable father. That cost is paid in relinquished autonomy. Parents want to control children; therefore they communicate that "father knows best, will make the decisions, and will tell you what to do." The price is commitment to patients, since fathers require the basic commitment to be to them and dutiful daughters comply; the price is creative role innovation because creative role innovation may mean departure for present roles. The price is too high.

"Woman's place is in the home," in the kitchen, and with the children. Woman's place is subordinate to men. The nurse's place is in the hospital, at the desk, and in the patient's room, following physician's orders. Nurse's place is subordinate to physicians.

Indeed, this is not true. The nurse's place is with the patient. The nurse is the patient's helper. The relationship between physician and nurse will be a healthy relationship when it is a colleagueship, mutually interdependent, and mutually helpful and supplementary and when it involves working, not in competition, but in collaboration for the benefit of the client. It is not the physician who will not allow the nurse to do this. Power is not taken from nurses by physicians; it is surrendered by nurses. The blaming of men and physicians is part of the victim-persecutor-rescuer game. Nurses must find their own level of autonomy and identity and begin to enact the roles they choose. Physicians will enact the complementary role as soon as the nurse evidences the benefit to the patient. Primary nurses have greater success in enacting colleagueship-type roles than do other nurses, probably because the benefits are so obvious that people in complementary roles see and enjoy those benefits.

MEDICAL CONTROL OF HEALTH CARE DELIVERY SYSTEMS

Basically the control of health care delivery systems by physicians has two results that influence nursing.

The first is the use of the medical model almost exclusively in dealing with patients. Medicine has traditionally been divided into specialty areas, according to convenient ways of educating physicians. Medical specialty areas can be according to physiological system, such as obstetrics-gynecology, orthopedics, cardiology, and neurology. Division can also be according to the type of treatment necessary for dealing with a condition, thus resulting in medical or surgical specialties. Other divisions are based on patient age or developmental level, such as pediatrics or gerontology, or by the phase of care needed, such as prevention or rehabilitation. These specialities arose in response to developing scientific knowledge and the need to provide efficient patient care. Nursing and other health care giving agencies followed suit. Hospitals were built for the physicians' convenience, and patients were segregated by "service areas" such as orthopedics, gynecology, and others. Nursing state board examinations conform to the medical model of specialty area, and graduate education uses the same divisions. Almost all health care literature is written to conform to this model, which pervades all aspects of health care. Nursing care systems that respond to the patient as a holistic organism and thus view and respond to man as a unit are few. This is primarily a result of the unquestioning acceptance of the practice of fracturing care into the stages of illness, physiological system, and/or developmental level, which serves medicine. Nursing care systems that view and respond to (1) the total family, regardless of the age of its members, (2) the total person, regardless of his medical diagnosis or the physiological system involved, and (3) the total problem, regardless of whether it is predominantly preventive or rehabilitative will be viable alternatives to the fractured piecemeal care usually offered. Primary nursing offers such an alternative. Although born in acute care settings, it has counterparts and potentials for use in all nursing arenas and will, when further developed, be a way to deliver holistic nursing care.

The second outcome of the medical control of health care is the "gatekeeper" role of the physician. Norris[1] states: "Except in rare instances, everyone—patient and professional alike—must wait until the physician has seen the patient." The physician controls entry into and progress through the health care system. Thus far the physician has maintained control with support from society, legislators, and fellow professionals and is the only person who can propel the patient into and through the multidisciplinary, multileveled complex called "health care." Until nurses are able, like other professionals such as lawyers, dentists, and clergymen, to have direct access to patients and patients are able to have direct access to nurses, no true antonomy or true freedom of professional growth is possible. If this does not occur, nursing will never attain full professionalism. Agencies that have used nurses as primary care agents have found that patients will indeed respond to nurses on a direct access basis by choice. The nurse then refers the patient, when necessary, to the physician; similarly, the physician in this type of situation refers patients to nurses.[2]

One difficulty inherent in the physician-controlled system (the "gatekeeper" phenomenon) is that it works to keep the focus of health care on the symptoms and on the patient's responses to those symptoms and not on the total patient or the context of those symptoms. Symptoms are only a part of the whole patient; his whole response to problems, his life, his world, and his family affect his responsiveness to health problems and affect the way in which health problems are manifested, perceived, interpreted, and treated. As long as nurses have a narrow view of the patient, that is, one affected by disease-oriented medical models, and as long as nurses allow patient access to be controlled by others, nursing will offer inadequate services to patients.

NEEDS OF THE CLIENT AND THE SOCIAL SYSTEM

Nursing care systems usually flourish for some time before their adequacies and inadequacies become evident. Nursing usually starts with selection of an alternative and implementation of that alternative without any test of the system's serviceability except its pragmatic utilization. If in the judgment of the administration a system is effective, the system is supported by the nursing administration. A list of criteria for judging the effectiveness of a system is often incomplete, since the criteria do not relate to the total needs of the client system. Cost effectiveness and task accomplishment efficiency have most often been the two main criteria against which a nursing care system is measured. The development of a more complete set of criteria to judge nursing care delivery systems will enable nurses to test these systems more meaningfully and thereby determine whether a system has the potential for meeting the care needs of a particular clientele within a specific agency structure or nursing care setting. This will add a second dimension to the utilitarian aspect of evaluation and should make both potential strengths and liabilities evident from the beginning.

A close look at the social system in the United States and a concomitant look at the needs of the individual who is both a product and a supporter of this system can be means for devising a beginning list of criteria to measure a nursing care delivery system's effectiveness.

The social system has several dominant characteristics that are reflected in the needs of patients. These patient needs provide criteria for measuring a nursing care delivery system. The social system in the United States is characterized by (1) the democratic process, (2) affluence, (3) mobility, (4) literacy, (5) social and cultural diversity, (6) belief in the power of American technology and ingenuity, (7) mechanization and automation of the environment, (8) increasing humanism, and (9) materialism.

The democratic process. The democratic process is characterized by two elements: authority vested in a leader by consent of the public and an educated electorate. Both these characteristics have implications for nursing. The democratic system gave rise to bureaucracy. The conflict between democracy and bureaucracy is a deep one, but the two systems seem to thrive on one another. In the bureaucratic system, leadership is imposed whereas in the democratic system, leaders are supposedly chosen. The basis of democracy rests in freedom of choice, and this concept is applied in health care in the following manner: freedom to choose a leader is similar to the freedom to choose one's own physician; freedom to impeach or fire that leader is similar to the freedom to leave the care of a chosen physician. The limitation by society of the freedom to choose a health *leader* (that is, a primary care giver) is inherent in the "gatekeeper" power currently granted to physicians. The bureaucratic system of supervisory control conflicts with the democratic ideal of freedom of choice, especially if translated into limited access to health care givers. The primary need of patients reflected in the democratic process is the need to choose the care giver who can best meet the patient's own perceived needs at that time. CRITERION: *Direct access of clients to care givers and access of care givers to clients, regardless of the titles of those health care givers.*

The educational level of the population is a direct outgrowth of the democratic form of government. Democracy requires an informed electorate so that wise choices can be made. In France and England as well as in the United States the principle of an informed electorate gave birth to free public schools. Virtually all democratic countries have systems of free public schools. Countries in which autocracy was the form of government were slower to educate the common man. The basic premise of the educated electorate is that education prepares an individual for the participatory governance that is the ideal of Jeffersonian democracy. This ideal is the basis for the patient's need for participation in his own health care. Never before in history has the layman been so well informed about health. Newspaper articles, regular health columns, family-oriented magazines, television reports, and school courses are geared to health and have succeeded in enabling patients to participate in their own assessment, diagnosis, and treatment. Patients can and do participate in the preventive, treatment, and rehabilitative aspects of care in a way never before possible, and are continually demanding increasing participation in their health care. CRITERION: *Equal participation by clients and care givers in all aspects of health care.*

Affluence. The United States is predominantly an affluent country. Not only are the middle classes fairly affluent, but also the poverty-level classes have a certain solvency when considered in relationship to many other countries of Western civilization. However, starvation and hopeless poverty do exist in this country. There is a widening gap between the rich and the poor, and there is every indication of increasing poverty as inflation accelerates. On the whole, however, American life is affluent. Affluence leads to sophistication regarding efficiency and cost effectiveness. Spiraling inflation in the cost of being ill and preventing illness has alerted the health care consumer to wasteful practices. The health care client needs and demands an efficient and effective system of nursing care that is also cost effective. CRITERION: *An efficient, effective nursing care delivery system that is cost effective without jeopardizing safety while increasing quality.*

Mobility. The American is characteristically mobile. Although migration was once considered a function of migrant farm workers only, many other occupations are now based on the concept of mobilization of personnel. Workers who are obviously mobile such as salesmen, airline crews, and entertainers are, surprisingly, in the minority. Companies having divisions in most of the states comprise a larger group; for example, General Electric, General Motors, International Business Machines, Standard Oil, and other major businesses transfer personnel from area to area and contribute large numbers of people to the migrant population. The most mobile, however, are those people who work in businesses that do not provide such benefits as job security or "tenure." These are skilled and semi-skilled workers who can market their talents in any section of the country, such as tradespeople, auto mechanics, hairdressers, carpenters, steel workers, farm laborers, waitresses, day laborers, etc. These people can and do move from place to place, following their own private star. Climate, better salaries, availability of a particular sport, relatives, or any number of other factors motivate mobility. If plotted on a map, this movement would be represented by a picture of constant circular activity.

Even more mobile is the population within a specific area. People frequently move within a twenty-five- to fifty-mile radius. They move from a larger to a smaller house, or vice versa, as the family expands or decreases. People change jobs in the same community and move closer to their work. They either become more or less affluent and move to reflect these financial status changes. People tire of yard work and maintenance of homes and move to apartments or conversely tire of having no yard and move from apartments to homes. Reasons for moving are as varied as the movers themselves.

The situation of concern here is that patients are mobile, and this mobility causes a fragmentation of health care. Continuity of care is almost impossible unless the client chooses to continue the nurse-patient relationship. Patients move around but may or may not change their physician, depending on how far they move from his location. However, if they do stay within a fifty-mile radius, they probably maintain their personal physician contact. This is because the patient wants and needs continuity of care. Continuity is important in meeting the holistic patient needs and responding to these needs as they fluctuate along the health-illness continuum. Patients go back to their original physician because they think he knows them and cares about them and because he has a complete history of their physical health.

The nurse also needs continuity. Nurses work with a client for days, weeks, or months and invest much of self. Too often patients disappear. They may be discharged or transferred, they may die, or they may move to another location; therefore the nurse does not have a sense of completion. There is limited feedback about the effectiveness of nursing care and little opportunity to observe a patient long enough to make meaningful adjustments to nursing plans. Feedback is essential to growth and care improvement. Continuity provides an opportunity to obtain such feedback. CRITERION: *Continuity of patient care that is not geographically based to home, hospital, or work setting but encompasses all settings and can be communicated to other nurses when patients move to different geographical areas.*

Literacy. The typical American is literate. He reads, he writes, and he is somewhat informed about health care and health needs. He reads *Today's Health* while waiting to see his physician. He reads the dental magazines when waiting to see his dentist. The middle-class American subscribes to *Psychology Today, Scientific American, Reader's Digest,* and other magazines. The housewife buys *Woman's Day* at the grocery store, and the young businessman reads *Penthouse* and *Playboy*. All these magazines, every newspaper, and every television station carry health-oriented information. Every magazine and television station advertises patent medicines. Health is a multibillion dollar industry, and since Americans are literate, they are increasingly aware that the key to health is not necessarily in cures but in prevention. Tons of vitamins are sold annually, health food stores are flourishing across the nation, and spas are making a fortune. Joggers jog, cyclers cycle, and swimmers swim. Americans are bent on low-cholesterol intake, motivated by the desire for longevity, and the key is prevention. The literate American wants and needs a nursing care system that prevents poor health as a primary focus and concentrates on care-cure when prevention fails or is not possible. CRITERION: *Prevention-oriented care that provides the care-cure and rehabilitative aspects of nursing care when prevention fails or is not possible.*

Social and cultural diversity. The United States has one of the most ethnically diverse populations in the world. Many countries have diverse populations as a result of mobility, but because the United States is so vast geographically and for many years had fairly open immigration laws, ethnic diversity is common even in the central states. Although not a product of immigration, Afro-Americans make up a significant percentage of the American population. Spanish-speaking Americans make up another significant percentage. Large ethnic populations of Polish, Irish, European Jews, Germans, and Scandinavians are scattered around the nation. On the West Coast and in New York are large populations of Chinese and Japanese Americans. In addition, pockets of religious and ethnic groups have existed in the country for two or three hundred years. The Amish and the Mennonites are examples of these ethnic groups. Finally, there are tribes of native American Indians. Few states do not have one or more tribes of Indians residing within their borders. Since the United States has no state religion but rather religious freedom, a wide variety of religions coexist nationwide. Religious diversity goes beyond the three commonly accepted major religions of Western civilization—Judaism, Catholicism, and Protestantism: it extends to Hinduism, Krishnaism, the Black Muslim religion, Islam, Buddhism, Taoism, and others. The need exists therefore for the patient to have care that responds to his ethnicity and to him as a member of a family and a community. For families have their dynamics, with their roles and relationships molded by the ethnic background of its members. Communities are comprised of families that congregate for mutual protection, welfare, and education, as well as cooperative sustenance. The needs of the individual client for nursing care that responds to his ethnic diversity is the beginning of the family-community health needs picture. CRITERION: *Responsiveness to the client in the context of his social and ethnic uniqueness as part of a family and a community.*

Belief in the power of American technology and ingenuity. Americans are so technologically oriented and their belief in the ability of American technology to master all problems is so great that it is difficult for them to imagine a problem to which science and technology cannot be applied to obtain an answer. Thus all health problems including incurable diseases and terminal conditions are viewed as temporary problems that scientists will solve eventually. Indeed, part of this American belief continues to be reinforced by the simple fact that scientific knowledge and medical and pharmacological discoveries are increasing at a high rate. Every time a major health problem is overcome by research and technology, belief in American technology is reinforced. Polio, tuberculosis, and measles vaccines; antibiotics such as penicillin and tetracycline; the heart-lung machine, replacement valves for the heart, Dacron blood vessel replacements, the dialysis procedure, and other advancements have all played their part in reinforcing the idea that American scientists are able to master any problem that arises in the health care field.

Another fact has not escaped the public: many major scourges of the past and, indeed, of recent years have been overcome or controlled by preventive medicine. Major plagues that once decimated the world, such as yellow fever, malaria, bubonic plague, smallpox, polio, and rabies, are but a few of the health problems that have been controlled by preventive medicine. Prevention may be the result of a vaccine or because of a vector control program. A disease may be locally controlled as malaria is controlled in the United States or controlled worldwide as in the case of smallpox, but prevention has proved to be the most effective cure. Americans believe, with some substantial reasons, that advancing science and technology will cure all; they feel that cancer and heart disease will be curable in the near future. For this reason, patients seek and need the most scientifically advanced and technologically current nursing care available. Skill is expected to accompany scientific knowledge. Educational prestige is tied to skill. Americans expect and need the most highly skilled delivery of care possible. CRITERION: *Technologically current and scientifically advanced care delivered with skill.*

Mechanization and automation of the environment. Modern man lives in a milieu that is mechanized and automated. His bills are sent by computer, and the checks he uses for paying bills are cleared by machine. Parking is monitored by meter, and food can be procured from vendors. Electric eyes open doors, closed circuit televisions monitor banks, and escalators and self-operated elevators move passengers from floor to floor. Automated Santas say "ho, ho, ho," and automated angles sing with the voices of the Mormon Tabernacle Choir. Anyone who has every tried, without success, to confront a computer with an incorrect monthly billing statement knows about the frustration and hopelessness resulting from the effort as well as the impersonality with which needed adjustments are ignored. The human voice on the telephone states that the problem is taken care of, but the bills keep showing the enormous charges. The computer "monkey" sees no changes, hears no changes, and computes no changes. Food vending machines provide hot coffee, hot soup, sandwiches, pies, and toothpicks but no conversation, no smile, and no thought for the day. Electric eye door openers do not say "good morning" or greet an individual by name. True, they require no tips, but that now seems small payment for a real relationship. Automated Santas do not really care what is wanted for Christmas, and the Mormon Tabernacle angels' speaker gets a buzz in it.

Patients receive impersonal treatment from machines. It is true that machines are not prejudiced and provide the same services to all, regardless of race, color, sex, or creed. One does feel rather silly, on the other hand, loving and hating a machine. People are important parts of an individual's daily life. Strangers can be meaningful to each other in chance encounters. Isolation and impersonality corrode the fabric of reality and can themselves be causes of health problems. Patients need personal, individualized nursing care that has special human elements and warm relationships as implicit and explicit components. CRITERION: *Personal, individualized nursing that is warm and caring.*

Increasing humanism. Perhaps in response to automation or perhaps in a maturing of the human state, man is becoming more widely humanistic. People are more conscious of social injustice and more active in its eradication. People are more alert to the needs of others and more willing to work singly and collectively to alter others' unhappy states. Despite pockets of evidence to the contrary, generally, man is seeing himself and his neighbors more and more as total humans, with real and meaningful responses to stimuli. The splitting of man into parts, by using terms such as soul, brain, physical, and emotional, is increasingly intolerable to a literate public who knows that the total child responds to poor parenting and that there is no purely "emotional" problem without all the other "parts" of the person responding also. Humans as holistic entities respond organismically to stimuli. There is no alteration of one part that does not affect the whole. The fallacy to date has been that scientists in studying the parts have not realized that the sum of those parts does not equal the whole. The whole is different from the total of the parts because of the unique way each individual is "wired." Humanism as such reflects a belief in the holistic nature and the dynamic aspects of life. Humanists believe life is a process; therefore it is never static but always growing and evolving. Conditions in the environment of man, such as human relationships and the conditions under which people live and are treated, affect the growth process and therefore the total health of the individual. Safety has become a description of totality, not just physical protection from harm. Safety is protection from harm or damage in any way and includes all the "parts." However, protection of any part must not jeopardize the integrity and safety of the total organism. Man, as a result of the rising consciousness and enactment of humanism, requires safe care in all aspects of his being, care that is delivered to him either comprehensively or organismically. CRITERION: *Safe care delivered organismically (comprehensively).*

Materialism. Materialism is characteristic of Americans in spite of increasing evidence that there is a rebellion against materialism. Creature comforts, luxury items, possession of vacation property and equipment, multiple automobiles, and multiple television sets mark the middle-class family. Lower income families strive to make enough money to improve their collection of comfort and luxury items. Some people decry materialism as corrosive to the moral system of America, and others value it for its ability to motivate work and productive activity. Regardless of value judgments, materialism exists as a major characteristic of the American social system. Most Americans are motivated by materialistic rewards. They enjoy material possessions, frequent luxury motels when they travel, admire luxurious houses and public buildings, and, in general, get a sense of security and well-being from the material comforts of life. Patients need and want a nursing care system that provides a comfortable environment, with as much attention to the luxuries as possible. CRITERION: *Attention to the comfort and luxuriousness of the health care environment.*

Criteria for Optimum Care System

A good nursing care delivery system, then, should meet the following criteria:
1. Direct access of clients to care givers and access of care givers to clients regardless of the titles of those health care givers
2. Equal participation by clients and care givers in all aspects of health care
3. An efficient, effective nursing care delivery system that is cost effective without jeopardizing safety while increasing quality
4. Continuity of patient care that is not geographically based to home, hospital, or work setting but encompasses all settings and can be communicated to other nurses when patients move to different geographical areas
5. Prevention-oriented care that provides the care-cure and rehabilitative aspects of nursing care when prevention fails or is not possible
6. Responsiveness to the client in the context of his social and ethnic uniqueness as part of a family and a community
7. Technologically current and scientifically advanced care delivered with skill
8. Personal, individualized nursing that is warm and caring
9. Safe care delivered organismically (comprehensively)
10. Attention to the comfort and luxuriousness of the health care environment

SUMMARY AND IMPLICATIONS FOR NURSING

The challenge. To have a system of care that meets the previously listed criteria, nurses must continue to work at creating innovative delivery systems. However, nurses need rewards and satisfactions from their work to continue the growing creative process of devising new and better modes of care. Rewards for nurses come from seeing patients respond to their care. Therefore continuity becomes important to nursing satisfaction.

Nurses need a sense of completion of a task. The fracturing of nursing care components in the functional method left nurses with little bits and pieces of care and no sense of the whole. The totality of the picture, the wholeness of the patient in the context of his family and his community, and the realness of his individuality and uniqueness were often missed in any system of care that omitted comprehensiveness. Therefore nurses not only need to see the task through to completion, but they need to see the whole task.

Nurses need a sense of autonomy, that is, a sense of being responsible and accountable for the assessment, planning, and delivering of care. They want to choose the person who will be their validator, consultant, and quality-control source for patient care. Autonomy and direct access are Siamese twins. Each is intertwined with the other, and if one is to live, the other must also thrive.

Nurses need a sense of authority so that decisions made, plans devised, and care prescribed can be implemented. Authority or power to act comes with autonomy, and one does not come without the other. Authority is not only the ability to carry out plans of care but also involves being accountable for those acts and their successes and failures. Authority and accountability provide nurses with motivation to do better quality work. They are perhaps the most motivating factors in learning, in growing, and in developing skills to levels of increasing competence.

Nurses need financial and material security. Financial and material security are rewards for difficult tasks that are successfully completed. Nurses need recognition from employers for the quality work performed by them. They can no longer be satisfied with low wages, a result of employers' excuses that nurses provide only second incomes and "family supplements," they must be awarded both salary levels and fringe benefits given men in positions requiring comparable education and comparable skills.

Any nursing care situation that does not meet the needs of nurses will not succeed as a system. The system and the agency or employing mechanism through which the system flows must be altered for that nursing care delivery package to endure and succeed.

To meet these criteria of a successful system and the needs of nurses, nursing and nurses must undergo many changes. Some implications of these changes are as follows:

1. Nursing must increase its level of awareness of the missing developmental level of autonomy and make conscious and concerted efforts to complete that developmental task.
2. Nurses must develop a clear view of the influence of business and industrial models of administration and production on nursing. They must begin to develop critical looks at the strengths and liabilities of such models to meet nursing care needs of clients.
3. Nursing must view its own needs as legitimate and understand that its needs are not necessarily antithetical to patient needs. Furthermore, nurses must learn that by meeting their own needs they often improve their ability to meet the needs of clients. More than that, nurses' needs and clients' needs are often so similar that they can be met with some of the same measures.
4. Nurses must become more aware of the social mores and folkways about women and refuse to play roles that reinforce a system in which both nursing and clientele suffer as a consequence. Nurses must work at being colleagues to other health care givers and must be committed to nursing as an important part of life.
5. Nurses must have more up-to-date knowledge about advancements in both

biological and social sciences so that they can utilize these advances in implementing nursing care.

6. Nursing personnel from the staff nurse level through the nursing director level must be retrained so that managerial functions alter, thus enabling direct care functions and systems to alter in ways that are more responsive to the needs of society, clients, and nurses.

7. Nurses must gain practice in colleagueship. They must learn to utilize each other in roles of peer validation, peer quality control, and peer mutual accountability. Valuing an associate's talents and expertise and using the associate as a consultant may be difficult for the nurse, but it is necessary to a nursing care delivery system that hopes to succeed.

The response. When the nursing care system responds to the following needs, then nursing will have devised a nursing care system that meets the criteria discussed previously:

1. The client's needs first and then, by way of the client, the needs of total families and total communities for comprehensive health care on a continuing basis

2. The nurse's needs for a sense of success with care, daily growth, autonomy, authority, and accountability

3. The need to attain the developmental level of maturity for the profession, having attained autonomy and marked by generativity and integrity in its care delivery system

4. The needs for nursing care that arise out of the social context of the country, made viable by awareness of that context

Primary nursing has been a giant step in the direction of response to these needs. Primary nursing care offers nursing a model. The model will grow and alter in the next few years as trial and validation and feedback and restructuring take place. However, the major step has been taken. Primary nursing offers a way to provide quality care that includes continuity and comprehensiveness for the patient; autonomy, authority, and accountability for the nurse; and an efficient, cost-effective system for the health care agency and for society.

REFERENCES

1. Norris, Catherine M.: Direct access to the patient, American Journal of Nursing **70:**1006-1007, 1970.
2. Armor, Nancy: The nurse practitioner at Kaiser Hospital, a speech delivered at the Sigma Theta Tau meeting, 1970.

SUGGESTED READINGS

Alexander, Edyth L.: Nursing administration in the hospital health care system, St. Louis, 1972, The C. V. Mosby Co.

Bennis, Warren G., Benne, Kenneth, and Chin, Robert: The planning of change, ed. 2, New York, 1972, Holt, Rinehart & Winston, Inc.

Berne, Eric.: Games people play, New York, 1964, Grove Press.

Bullough, Vern L., and Bullough, Bonnie: The emergence of modern nursing, ed. 2, New York, 1969, The Macmillan Co.

Colwill, Jack M.: The shifting emphasis in the delivery of health care: viewpoint of a physician. In Primary health care: everybody's business, Publication No. 20-1482, New York, 1973, National League for Nursing, pp. 9-19.

Cumbie, Charlotte: The shifting emphasis in the delivery of health care: viewpoint of a nurse. In Primary health care: everybody's business, Publication No. 20-1482, New York, 1973, National League for Nursing, pp. 32-35.

Durbin, Richard L., and Sprengall, W. Herbert: Organization and administration of health care: theory, practice, environment, St. Louis, 1969, The C. V. Mosby Co.

Gilbert, Albert F.: Managing change in the hospital, Hospital Topics **47**:40-41, July, 1969.

Glaser, William A.: Nursing leadership and policy: some cross-national comparisons. In Davis, Fred, editor: The nursing profession: five sociological essays, New York, 1966, John Wiley & Sons, Inc., pp. 1-59.

Goode, William J.: The theoretical limits of professionalization. In Etzioni, Amitai, editor: The semi-professions and their organization. New York, 1969, The Free Press, pp. 266-313.

Graves, Helen Hope: Can nursing shed bureaucracy? American Journal of Nursing **70**:490-494, 1971.

Knecht, Aileen Atwood: Innovation on Four Tower West: why? American Journal of Nursing **73**:809-810, 1973.

Kramer, Marlene: Team nursing: a means or an end? Nursing Outlook **19**:648-652, 1971.

Kramer, Marlene: Nursing care plans: power to the patient, Journal of Nursing Administration, pp. 29-34, Sept.-Oct., 1972.

Levin, Pamela, and Berne, Eric: Games nurses play, American Journal of Nursing **72**:483-487, 1972.

Lewis, Edith P.: Editorial: a nurse is a nurse—or is she? Nursing Outlook **20**:21, 1972.

Lombertsen, Eleanor C.: Nursing team organization and function, New York, 1953, Columbia University Press.

McCormack, Regina C., and Crawford, Ronald L.: Attitudes of professional nurses toward primary care. In Lewis, Edith P.: Changing patterns of nursing practice: new needs, new roles, New York, 1971, The American Journal of Nursing Co., pp. 124-129.

Manthey, Marie, and Kramer, Marlene: A dialogue on primary nursing between Marie Manthey and Marlene Kramer, Nursing Forum **9**:356-379, 1971.

Maubach, Hans O.: The organizational context of nursing practice. In Davis, Fred, editor: The nursing profession: five sociological essays, New York, 1966, John Wiley & Sons, Inc., pp. 109-137.

Rogers, Martha E.: Nursing: to be or not to be? Nursing Outlook **20**:43-46, Jan., 1972.

Schlegel, Margaret Werner: Innovation on Four Tower West: how? American Journal of Nursing **73**:811-813, 1973.

Schutt, Barbara G.: Spot check on primary care nursing, American Journal of Nursing **72**:1996-2003, 1972.

Seward, Joan F.: Professional practice in a bureaucratic structure, In Lewis, Edith P.: Changing patterns of nursing practice: new needs, new roles, New York, 1971, The American Journal of Nursing Co., pp. 37-44.

Thompson, Victor A.: Hierarchy, specialization, and organizational conflict, Administrative Science Quarterly **5**:486-521, 1961.

Wolford, H.: Complemental nursing care and practice, Nursing Forum **3**:8-20, 1964.

Young, Lucie S.: Needs of the patient as seen by the nurse, In Auld, Margaret E., and Birum, Linda Hulthen, editors: The challenge of nursing, St. Louis, 1973, The C. V. Mosby Co., pp. 17-23.

II

THE NATURE AND SCOPE
OF PRIMARY NURSING

chapter 3

PRIMARY NURSING AS EMPLOYED IN VARIOUS SETTINGS THROUGHOUT THE COUNTRY

The public, whether called patients or clients, is demanding health care services that are more reflective of its needs. In some cases these new services are vastly different from traditional approaches to health care delivery. The high cost to the patient for outdated, often mediocre services is prompting government officials at all levels to take a new look at providing higher quality coverage to patients at prices they can afford. Although the emphasis to provide patients with quality, individual, and comprehensive nursing services is still largely in the community, hospitals too are reevaluating the nursing services they provide to patients. Hospitals are realizing that if they do not "get on the bandwagon," patient's increasing ability to choose services will put those failing to provide high-quality care out of the market.

Nurse practitioners, primex nurses, and independent group practitioners are some of the nursing roles that have been developed to provide primary care to patients in the community setting. Primary nurses are their counterpart in the hospital setting, but they differ from these other practitioners in that primary nurses may view the patient more comprehensively and could be involved past the primary care stages.

In the following discussion these new roles will be described and compared to provide a clearer conception of what is happening with nursing modalities around the country and in various settings. Also, a review of how primary nursing is being utilized will be presented.

INDEPENDENT NURSE ROLES

Many nurses have become independent practitioners and have taken their rightful place as peers of the physicians in the community. Nurse practitioners are reaching out to the public and are assuming the active, accountable, and highly responsible role of providing primary care to clients.[1]

Primex, primary care, or primary care nursing refers to nurses who provide assessment and care at an initial point in the patient's illness as a preventive measure or to maintain the present health status. Secondary nursing care refers

39

to services provided to patients or clients after they have entered a health care delivery system in which the focus is on restorative and maintenance services.[2] Primary nursing refers to nurses in the hospital or secondary setting who provide the initial patient assessment and assume accountability for planning comprehensive twenty-four–hour care for an individual patient for the duration of hospitalization and immediately thereafter. At the same time the primary nurse provides nursing care services to the patient and coordinates the care with associate nurses.

Independent nurse roles in the community and the hospital emphasize the health and wellness of patients, foster coordination and continuity of care, and provide comprehensive services to the patient. Furthermore, nurses who assume independent roles have the opportunity to practice nursing in a highly professional way.

In addition to making the initial health assessment, nurse practitioners or primex nurses coordinate all aspects of the patient's health and life-style in the community. They make referrals and collaborate with physicians and other health disciplines. Continuity of care is provided to patients within and between health services. Independent nurse practitioners keep their knowledge regarding preventive illness and maintenance of health care programs current. They are also adaptable and flexible so that they can adapt to meet future health needs.

Independent group practitioners might function in a similar way to nurse practitioners but utilize a team concept. The team would be comprised of a team leader who is a registered nurse (R.N.) with a baccalaureate degree in nursing, registered nurses from other training programs, licensed vocational nurses (L.V.N.s), aides, and community health workers as team members. The group practice would be community based and usually located in a vicinity near physicians' offices or purveyors of secondary health care services. The team would be directly associated with one or more physicians.

These group practitioners, as conceived by Murray,[3] make primary health contacts and initial patient assessments, including family histories, with data about psychosocial aspects, coping mechanisms, health and illness experiences, and life-style patterns. Identifying deviations from healthy physical or behavioral functioning and counseling on nonacute health problems are functions of the team. In addition, the team provides education to individuals and groups concerning maintenance of their own health and prevention of illness as well as assists patients to obtain medical care as needed.

The community nursing team initiates and follows through on physician's orders related to diagnosis and treatment and works collaboratively with other health professionals to coordinate the total health care for individual patients. The team further initiates and provides supervision for rehabilitative measures for patients with chronic illnesses and disabilities.

Hospital-based independent nurses, or primary nurses, also assume an active, accountable, and highly responsible role in providing health care services to patients. Within the hospital setting, primary nurses make initial patient assessments; initiate a twenty-four–hour nursing care plan based on data obtained from the patient, his family, and physician; and coordinate all aspects of the patient's care during hospitalization. The primary nurse, as the liaison person between hospital and community, recommends to and counsels the patient about community resources and most often follows up the patient in his home immediately after discharge from the hospital.

Primary nursing differs from other hospital health care delivery systems in that it promotes individualized patient care or peer and colleague relationships with co-workers, physicians, supervisors, and other health workers. Primary nurses practice the art and science of nursing, make nursing judgments and decisions, and accept responsibility for those decisions. They collaborate with other professionals who are providing services to an individual patient. Nursing leaders such as supervisors and head nurses assume consultant and resource functions for primary nurses.

A DESCRIPTION OF PRIMARY NURSING IN SETTINGS ACROSS THE COUNTRY

The reasons for selecting primary nursing as a patient care delivery system are many, according to several hospitals surveyed. Agencies point out the ever-growing concern by hospital administrators and practicing nurses that hospitalized patients need higher quality, more individualized services.

Although many hospitals have accepted the challenge of implementing primary nursing, the growth of primary nursing is still in the infant stage across the country. Not all hospitals are experimenting with this form of nursing care delivery. However, in those hospitals that are seeing positive results soon after implementation of the new system, motivation for its use is high. The few hospitals that are experimenting seem to be satisfied to just achieve a different organizational way of providing patient care services, culminating in a case method approach. These hospitals will be satisfied with their halfway adaptation to the criteria.

Those hospitals that have progressed the most are implementing primary nursing to achieve more individualized patient care services and are also aiming to employ roles and organizational features that enhance primary nursing. If implemented correctly, the process of primary nursing lends itself to flexibility, creativity, and innovation. These aspects of primary nursing make the system adaptable to individualized patient care and make it possible to foster other changes in patient care. It is important to remember that primary nursing, in addition to being a different way of organizing work, is more importantly a vehicle for hospitals and nurses to provide and extend care services that are individual and relevant to the patient. Primary nursing is also the vehicle that can allow nurses to work and develop at the highest professional level. This may prevent nurses from becoming disenchanted and leaving the hospital for places in which they perceive they can practice as "professional" nurses.

Numbers of hospitals implementing primary nursing. Of the ten hospitals surveyed and known to be experimenting with primary nursing, six are on the West Coast, two are in the Midwest, and two are on the East Coast. The units selected by the hospitals for the implementation of primary nursing are varied. They include pediatrics, respiratory, coronary care, intensive care, and medical-surgical units. The reasons for selecting particular units for primary nursing reflect staff attitudes and motivation on these units, as well as the type of patients housed on these units.

There does not seem to be a large-scale push to implement primary nursing throughout hospitals. Rather, nursing administrations are leaving the selection of the patient care delivery system up to the individual unit's staff. Head nurses and staff members are able to compare the different systems and make final decisions based on the philosophy and needs of the staff.

Criteria for selection of unit and staff. Head nurses on units selected for primary nursing are generally young, innovative, motivated, and highly patient care oriented. Although they do not participate directly in giving patient care, they see the importance of coordinating all aspects of patient care and staff development and act in consultative roles to staff. The head nurse usually interprets the system to physicians and other hospital departments and helps the staff develop their plans and ideas.

In almost all the hospitals surveyed, the head nurse is seen as the person who determines the unit climate and permits innovative nursing practice. The head nurses are responsible for the twenty-four–hour functioning and management of their units, whereas primary nurses assume accountability for direct patient care.

Nursing staff attitudes prior to primary nursing were generally task oriented. Although they gave safe and good care, staff nurses were not accustomed to a consistent plan for nursing care with a formal written care plan. Patient care was organized on a systematic basis and carried out in an efficient way for a given day. Although there is no argument with efficiency, staff nurses and patients alike remained unfulfilled. Staff nurses became aware of the need to decrease the fragmentation of care given to patients and regarded primary nursing as a way of achieving greater continuity and coordination of patient care. At the same time they perceived in primary nursing a way to develop and enhance their own abilities and maximize their professional commitment to nursing. Staff nurses on the primary nursing units surveyed were young, motivated, innovative, and accustomed to change. They considered the nursing process to be important and useful, and they were interested in improving the quality of patient care services. Two hospitals made a point of selecting staff nurses with these qualities to work on their primary nursing units.

Nurses on these units were expected to be clinically competent (not technically competent), to take nursing histories, to problem solve effectively, and to accept a new role of independence for planning and providing holistic patient care.

Some hospitals employed L.V.N.s as primary nurses, whereas other hospitals utilized them as associate nurses only. One unit in particular is presently training L.V.N.s to assume the primary nurse role. The L.V.N.s on this unit were able to identify their inadequacies for the role, but they expressed interest in developing and possibly assuming the role in the future.

In the hospitals surveyed, nurse's aides are not being used in either a primary or associate nurse capacity. Many hospitals are still unsure in what capacity to employ aides. Some hospitals are not utilizing them in any role on their primary nursing units. Still others are utilizing nurse's aides in a purely assisting capacity. Aides on these units are assisting other staff members as the need arises. They also pass water pitchers, take temperatures, make beds, and do many housekeeping chores.

Organization of primary nursing units. In primary nursing, a patient is assigned to a nurse based on the needs of the patient and the abilities and interests of the nurse. The head nurse is usually responsible for determining patient assignments.

Nurses on most primary nursing units provide "total patient care," although they may not identify themselves as primary and associate nurses. They also may not care for an individual patient for the duration of his hospitalization. In addition, the pairing of patient and nurse can be based on the unit geography. For example, a nurse is assigned to designated rooms, and the patients admitted to those rooms are automatically assigned to the nurse. In one hospital, nurses maintain a specific pediatric patient area for one month and then exchange geographical areas to work with different kinds of patients such as children of different ages on a pediatric unit. Another unit employs R.N.s as primary nurses who are responsible for several patients. The R.N. functions include writing nursing histories, initiation of written care plans, and medication regimens, as well as making rounds with the physician and with the L.V.N. and aide who will give the patient care.

A majority of these hospitals employ primary nurses on the day and evening shifts and associate nurses on all three shifts. Some units employ primary nurses on the day shift only. Primary nurses may have two or more patients, and associate nurses may have as many as four or more. Primary nurses function in both primary and associate nurse roles. For example, primary nurses working evenings can have three patients as a primary nurse and four patients as an associate nurse. The four "associate" patients have primary nurses who are on the day shift or on a day off. The night associate nurse, however, is considered a key factor in the twenty-four–hour communication of patient needs.

The typical staffing ratio on several units is as follows: days, five patients to one nurse; evenings, eight patients to one nurse; and nights, ten to thirteen patients to one nurse. On one unit surveyed, the ratio was nine to one, but an L.V.N. and aide provided the actual patient care to the nine patients.

Some units are utilizing a higher number of R.N.s on their primary nursing units, whereas others have not altered their ratio at all. Either way, hospitals agree that the primary nursing units are more cost-effective compared to their other units, even if the number of R.N.s has been increased.

Extended functions, such as home visits, physical examinations, and other services, can be initiated to enhance comprehensive and continuous patient care. Two hospitals have begun home visits, and several are allowing or considering allowing physical examinations by nurses. The ten-hour day is currently practiced in one hospital and under consideration by others. This lengthened shift is utilized to provide time for activities beyond the basic patient care activities, such as physical examinations, interviews, conferences, and others.

Reactions to the new system. The reaction to primary nursing by physicians, nursing staff, and nursing leaders has been largely highly favorable and positive. In one hospital, there was 100 percent agreement that primary nursing has resulted in better nursing care to patients.

Most physicians seem to agree that primary nurses are more insightful concerning patient needs. They see the benefits to their patients of direct communication, with primary nurses caring for their patients.

According to nurses and patients alike, a more in-depth relationship is one result of primary nursing. At the same time, trust is increasing in the nurse-patient relationship. It is common for the patient to identify the nurse as "my nurse" and for the nurse to identify the patient as "my patient."

Staff nurses are finding increased job satisfaction and increased respect for their profession because of primary nursing. They are able to utilize the nursing process and directly affect the course of patient care. Primary nurses across the country are motivated to accept the responsibility of providing and coordinating total, individualized patient care.

SUMMARY

Nurses in the community collaborate and work in colleague relationships with physicians and health services to provide comprehensive initial patient assessments, referrals to other agencies, and maintenance of present health status. As nurse practitioners, they are achieving the independence consistent with their educational level and, as a result, are professionally satisfied.

Hospital-based primary nurses are also emerging as collaborators and colleagues with physicians and personnel from other health disciplines. Primary nurses are assuming accountability for total, comprehensive patient care. They coordinate patient care and provide for continuity of care for the duration of hospitalization. In a similar way to nurse practitioners, primary nurses are achieving independence in the hospital setting throughout the country.

REFERENCES

1. Rogers, Martha E.: Nursing: to be or not to be? Nursing Outlook **20:**42-46, 1972.
2. Leininger, M. M., Little, D. E., and Carnevali, Doris: Primex, American Journal of Nursing **72:**1274-1277, 1972.
3. Murray, B. Louise: A case for independent group nursing practice, Nursing Outlook **20:**60-63, Jan., 1972.

SUGGESTED READINGS

Abdellah, F. G., Markin, A., Beland, I. L., and Matheny, R. V.: Patient-centered approaches to nursing, New York, 1961, The Macmillan Co.

Fagin, C. M., and Goodwin, G.: Baccalaureate preparation for primary care, Nursing Outlook **20:**240-244, April, 1972.

Schutt, B. G.: Spot check on primary care nursing, American Journal of Nursing **72:**1996-2003, 1972.

U. S. Department of Health, Education and Welfare: Extending the scope of nursing practice, Nursing Outlook **20:**46-52, 1972.

chapter 4

A MODEL FOR PRIMARY NURSING UNITS

Primary nursing is a mode of patient care delivery that bridges the gap between education and service and provides individualized care to patients. Primary nursing is the first nursing modality that nurses are taught. As students they select a specific number of patients, based on the patients' diagnosis or the students' focus. Students remain accountable for planning total, comprehensive patient care during hospitalization and after discharge from the hospital. They learn to interact and communicate effectively with physician, family, unit staff members, and hospital departments. They accept the responsibility for patient care and its follow through. Hospital resources become familiar to them, and they learn to use them effectively to coordinate their efforts for patient care.

Primary nursing is the way nursing "used to be" or "ought to be" for many patients. Patients remember when they had the same nurses taking care of them and that those nurses seemed to care about them. It has been documented that patients enter the hospital with apprehension, which can be relieved or may increase as the hospitalization continues. The primary nurse as the patient's advocate alleviates his anxiety. The whole patient—his life style, family interactions, medical history, occupation, religion, and expectations for this hospitalization—is the focus of the nurse. The patient is a person first, a person who has had his life interrupted by his illness and/or ensuing hospitalization. He generally looks forward to resuming a normal, healthy life but may be afraid of the consequences of this illness. Patients generally regard their life-styles as purposeful and special and hope that nurses caring for them will give them that consideration.

Primary nursing represents, in both theory and practice, an approach to patient care that emphasizes health and a sense of well-being. Nursing staff, physicians, and families concentrate on the preventive aspects as well as the therapeutic and restorative aspects of care.

PRIMARY NURSING OBJECTIVES

The objectives for a primary nursing unit emphasize staff development and promote a holistic approach to patient care. They communicate to staff, on a broad scale, what the expectations are for the unit. These objectives, as opposed to performance criteria, inform the individual staff member about the expectations for individual performance and inform the nurse about how the purpose of the unit will be fulfilled and what goals all staff have in common for the unit.

The key objective for a primary nursing unit is to provide optimum care and services to patients and their families by focusing nursing care on the individual patient's needs. Primary nursing as the main mode of distributing patient care responsibilities transcends the various levels of intervention, which are treatment, restoration, and prevention. Personal and professional development of the staff is an outgrowth of the nursing care modality of the unit.

Primary nurses become accountable for providing total, comprehensive, continuous, patient-centered care for the duration of the patient's hospitalization. Coordinating and communicating all aspects of patient care to physicians, families, and staff members become essential components of their accountability. More specifically, the unit objectives can be delineated to include the following guidelines for nursing staff:

A. Patient-centered care—to provide care in which the patient is the central focus for planning care, implementing care, and evaluating care
   1. To identify areas for nursing intervention, to assign priorities to these areas, and to develop a course of action that effectively meets the needs of the patient and family
   2. To initiate a written nursing care plan on admission by the primary nurse that includes a description of the patient's needs and problems, the assignment of priorities to these needs, consideration and discussion of multiple alternatives to meet these needs, a discussion of the consequences of each alternative solution, a decision to use one or more interventions, and a method of evaluating the results of the interventions
   3. To gather relevant data at the time of admission by obtaining a history and physical examination and data throughout the patient's hospitalization by means of patient and family interviews, observations, review of medical records, and professional consultations
   4. To reflect consideration of patient need areas, such as psychological, social, and physical needs, on the nursing care plan
B. Accountability for patient care—to assign staff and encourage the selection of patients by staff so that the most effective use is made of individuals' skills and knowledge through primary nursing, which is the assignment and accountability for the total nursing care of one patient and his family to a single nurse
   1. To provide for the selection of primary patients, based on capabilities of the nurse, needs of the patient and family, and the actual work to be done
   2. To promote evaluation of various methods of staff utilization that create the most effective means of scheduling nursing care and assigning nursing responsibilities for increasing nurse accountability and coordination of patient care

47

3. To accept the responsibility for total patient care planning, evaluating, and coordinating and communicating all aspects of patient-centered care to other health personnel and families so that continuity of care to the patient is enhanced

4. To include all staff members in the responsibility of continually assessing all nursing regulations so that the most appropriate and desirable standards are formulated for controlling and standardizing nursing care without violating hospital policies

C. Continuity of patient care—to provide for continuity of care by assigning one patient to one primary nurse who coordinates patient care and by selecting associate nurses who follow through on the plan of care

1. To ensure continuity of care by the assignment of a single nurse, that is, the primary nurse, to a single patient for the duration of the patient's hospitalization and by selection of associate nurses who follow through on the plan of care for the duration of the hospitalization

2. To continuously assess patient care needs and reflect this assessment in the care plan and to communicate this plan to others who are both directly involved and to those less intensively involved with the patient and his family

3. To communicate patient and family needs to other staff members during patient-centered conferences to promote a unified approach by staff for each individual patient

D. Comprehensive patient care—to provide a holistic approach to patient care as opposed to a specialized approach to patient care

1. To consider the emotional, psychosocial, spiritual, and physical aspects of patient problems and needs

2. To determine the type and amount of nursing care services needed (whether they involve prevention, restoration, or treatment) by extensive routine evaluations of patients and their families by their individual nurse

3. To include patients and their families in all aspects of planning and teaching, with consideration given to the individual patient's needs and his ability to assimilate information

4. To provide a humanistic approach to patient care in which the individual patient's needs and interests predominate in planning and implementing care

E. Coordination of patient care—to provide a congruous approach to patient care in which the more global aspects of care are highlighted

1. To effectively utilize the unit's personnel and physical resources for the development of staff and the improvement of patient care services and standards for care

2. To administer assistance and service to the patient and his family that are based on the nursing care plan and the physician's orders, with consideration given to alternative ways of providing each aspect of nursing care

3. To effectively utilize community resources as indicated throughout the patient's hospitalization and while planning for discharge and to coordinate this plan with the physician, patient, and patient's family

F. Staff development—to encourage and facilitate the growth and knowledge of the nursing staff by providing relevant learning opportunities

1. To measure the performance and attitudes of the nursing staff, using questionaires, interviews, and performance criteria
2. To maintain records of various innovations in nursing care and nursing policy
3. To improve individual performance by means of counseling and evaluations and by encouraging the nursing staff to independently identify their own problems and individual needs and to work together to enhance each others performance
4. To develop and utilize educational opportunities and resources in response to identified educational needs as they arise; these may involve in-service programs, workshops, individual supervision, and rotation through other shifts, nursing units, and positions
5. To encourage staff involvement in defining and evaluating educational programs for the unit and individual staff members
6. To provide an environment in which new concepts and ideas are fostered and in which nursing staff are encouraged to be creative in their thinking about the delivery of nursing care and the establishment of nursing procedures

PRIMARY NURSING UNIT ORGANIZATION

Unit organization and the lines of authority inherent in the organization need to be clearly defined for all nursing personnel. At the same time nursing staff involvement in describing the organizational structure can be encouraged to enhance staff understanding and support for the lines of authority. Fig. 4-1 shows the relationship between the director of nursing and the staff on a model primary nursing unit. The lines of authority are from the director to the head nurse and from the head nurse to the entire staff. The assistant head nurse and in-service coordinator are accountable to the head nurse but act in advisory roles to each other. The solid lines from the assistant head nurse and in-service coordinator indicate that when they act as replacements for the head nurse, they have authority over staff.

Because primary nursing encourages direct communication, it is important to create a horizontal hierarchy that can facilitate direct communication within the hierarchy. Fig. 4-2 is an example of the supervisor's relationship to the director of nursing and the head nurse. To eliminate the channels that often obstruct communication, the supervisor and head nurse are both directly accountable to the director but act in advisory, consultant, and complementary roles to each other. As a primary nursing care consultant, the supervisor will often confer with several units, providing clinical expertise and recommendations, but the head nurse

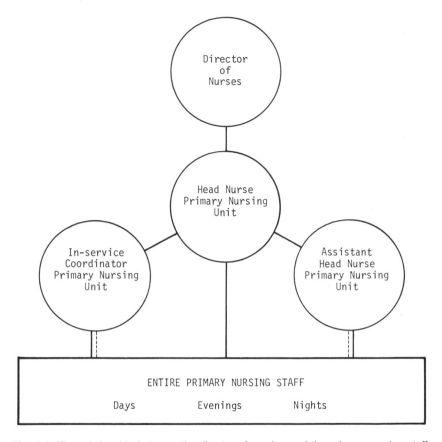

Fig. 4-1. The relationship between the director of nursing and the primary nursing staff.

remains directly accountable for the unit and needs an avenue of direct communication to the director of nurses.

The primary nurse as the patient's advocate is the hub of the wheel for all communications concerning the patient's care, the coordination of care throughout hospitalization, and the planning for discharge. Fig. 4-3 describes the relationship of the primary nurse and the patient to other health personnel, hospital departments, and community agencies.

Primary nurses communicate with associate nurses by means of nursing care plans, patient-centered conferences, and verbal communication. At the same time associate nurses can reflect changes in the patient's condition and needs on the nursing care plan and provide feedback to the primary nurse concerning assessments and observations of an individual patient.

The primary nurse recognizes that the family will play an important part in the patient's understanding and acceptance of his illness as well as in his overall re-

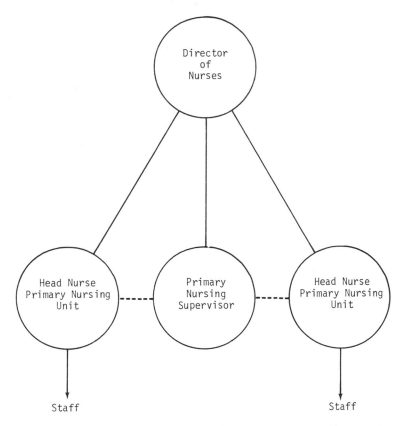

Fig. 4-2. The relationship between the director of nursing, primary nursing supervisor, and head nurses on primary nursing units.

covery. Therefore nurse-family interaction begins on admission of the patient. The family is told that they will be included in all teaching aspects of the patient's care. In-hospital family conferences can be held to discuss aspects of the patient's illness that may be unclear and to show the family how they can be supportive to the patient. Although families can contribute to the patient's sense of well-being during hospitalization, they can also detract from it by their own anxieties and lack of understanding. The primary nurse by counseling the family increases their understanding and promotes an anxiety-free environment for patient recovery.

The primary nurse's communication with hospital departments facilitates a greater understanding of the patient's needs by the departments and can help relieve the patient's anxieties during specific procedures. Because of this improved understanding, hospital personnel in various departments such as inhalation therapy, pharmacy, physical therapy, occupational therapy, and dietetics are

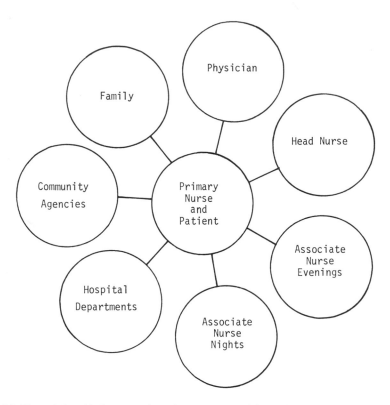

Fig. 4-3. The relationship between the primary nurse and the patient and others involved in his care.

better able to assist patients during treatments, with the fullest benefit to the patient.

Community agencies such as The American Heart Association, Diabetic Association, Cancer Society, and others can be excellent resources for community intervention while the patient is hospitalized. In addition, hospital social workers or public health nurses are excellent resources for primary nurses to collaborate with and coordinate community services during a patient's hospitalization and while planning for discharge.

The primary nurse, head nurse, and physician control the quality of care the patient receives by maintaining a daily feedback system. They are the three people directly accountable for the management of the patient's care. They meet routinely to discuss and agree on the rationale for care, to plan comprehensive care, to problem solve and to evaluate and coordinate patient care. The communication triangle in Fig. 4-4 represents the most important aspect of patient care management in a primary nursing setting. The triangle demonstrates the colleagueship between the head nurse, primary nurse, patient, and physician in

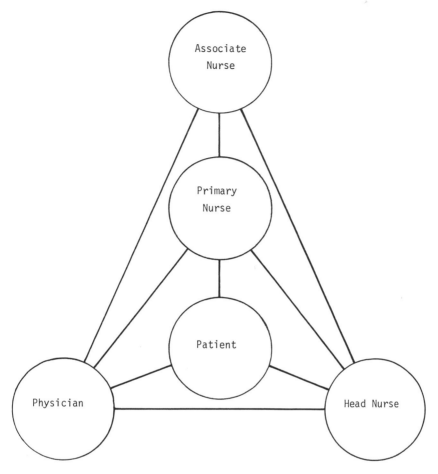

Fig. 4-4. Central communication triangle for primary nursing.

collaborating with each other and communicating information relevant to patient care planning, implementation, and evaluation. It also demonstrates that the patient is the center of focus for comprehensive planning of care.

Although not always involved in the direct communication, the head nurse continues to receive feedback from the physician or primary nurse concerning significant changes in planning, rationale, and treatment. The associate nurse in the primary nurse's absence enlarges the triangle and becomes an integral part of it and, like the head nurse, remains informed of the patient's management by communicating with the primary nurse. The primary nurse or associate nurse accompanies the physician on daily patient rounds to further coordinate care, enhance nursing intervention, and provide and receive validation and rationale for patient care management.

STAFF SCHEDULING

To effectively demonstrate primary nursing operationally, it is helpful to examine the structure of a model unit and the relationship of primary nurses to patients. In the model unit presented here, the staff will consist of only registered nurses. A model staff schedule is shown in Fig. 4-5 and demonstrates the scheduling of staff for all three shifts. This hypothetical unit has thirty beds and a full complement of twenty-three staff members. The distribution of staff for all three shifts is as follows:

SHIFT	STAFF MEMBERS	PATIENT ASSIGNMENTS
7 A.M. to 3:30 P.M.	6 to 8 on duty	4 to 6
3 A.M. to 11:30 P.M.	5 to 7 on duty	7 to 9
11 A.M. to 7:30 P.M.	2 to 4 on duty	9 to 15

The head nurse is not counted in the daily staffing on this schedule. Head nurses are accountable for the twenty-four–hour management of all the patients and the twenty-four–hour development of the entire staff. It is important that head nurses have flexible hours, such as 9 A.M. to 5:30 P.M., 6 A.M. to 2:30 P.M. or the full eight hours of any shift. In this way they will be free to meet with their evening and night shifts. In addition, their schedules must be flexible enough to allow them time off the unit to attend meetings as well as time for conferences, in-service meetings, and meetings on the unit. The head nurse on this schedule has every other weekend off. It should be noted that many hospitals are recognizing that the head nurse can be off every weekend or work only those weekends when surgeries, treatments, diagnostic tests, and other therapy is scheduled.

Flexibility of hours and rotation to other shifts by the head nurse promotes the continuous support to the staff that is necessary to ensure continuity of care to the patients. In the same way, shift rotation for staff nurses provides a global representation of the patient's needs and problems that will also ensure continuity of care.

Staff nurses can also be allowed flexibility of hours beyond shift rotation. Scheduling patterns of 8 A.M. to 4:30 P.M., 9 A.M. to 5:30 P.M., 2 A.M. to 10:30 P.M., and others can provide staff with the necessary time to do their patient's history and physicals, initiate care plans, interview patients, attend in-service conferences, etc. The organization of work can continue based on the 7:00 to 3:30 schedule, with other staff members assigned to maintain the overview of patient care until the 8:00 to 4:30 nurse arrives. From 3:30 to 4:30, this nurse is then free to pursue those activities that will contribute to assessment and comprehensive patient care. This type of scheduling can be employed on a rotational basis among staff members. Not shown on this schedule is the rotation expected between the in-service coordinator and the assistant head nurse. In complementary roles to the head nurse, they foster continuity and coordination of comprehensive patient care. To accomplish this, they also must maintain the twenty-four–hour overview of patient care and staff development.

A two-week rotation at the end of each six-week schedule is suggested. In-service coordinators working two weeks of evenings can evaluate the in-service

UNIT____________

	MARCH																														APRIL											
	S	M	T	W	Th	F	S	S	M	T	W	Th	F	S	S	M	T	W	Th	F	S	S	M	T	W	Th	F	S	S	M	T	W	Th	F	S	S	M	T	W	Th	F	S
DAYS	1	2	3	4	5	6	7	8	9	10	11	12	13	14	15	16	17	18	19	20	21	22	23	24	25	26	27	28	29	30	31	1	2	3	4	5	6	7	8	9	10	11
1A Head Nurse						X	X	X					X							X	X	X					X							X	X	X					X	
1B In-service Coor.	X	X							X					X	X	X							X					X	X	X							X					X
1C						X	X	X				X							X	X							X	X	X	X								X	X			
1D	X	X							X	X								X			X	X	X								X	X								X		X
1E				X	X								X	X	X				X						X	X								X	X	X					X	
1F						X	X	X				X						X	X								X	X	X				X						X	X		
1G	X	X								X	X						X				X	X	X								X	X						X				X
1H			X	X							X			X	X	X								X	X						X				X	X	X					
1I	X				X							X	X							X	X	X				X							X	X							X	X
1J			X	X						X				X	X	X								X	X					X					X	X	X					
1K			X				X	X	X								X	X						X				X	X	X								X	X			
EVENINGS																																										
2A Asst. H. N.	X	X							X					X	X	X							X					X	X	X							X					X
2B	X	X								X	X									X	X	X					X				X	X								X		X
2C						X	X	X				X				X	X							X				X	X	X								X	X			
2D				X	X								X	X	X				X							X	X							X	X	X					X	
2E	X	X								X	X							X			X	X	X								X				X	X	X					
2F						X	X	X				X								X	X	X				X							X	X							X	X
2G				X	X								X	X	X				X					X	X							X			X	X	X					
2H			X				X	X	X								X	X							X			X	X	X								X	X			
NIGHTS																																										
3A	X	X									X	X								X	X	X	X									X	X								X	X
3B						X	X	X	X									X	X								X	X	X	X									X	X		
3C			X	X									X	X	X	X									X	X								X	X	X	X					
3D						X	X						X	X						X	X						X	X						X	X						X	X
DAYS	6	7	7	7	8	7	6	6	7	7	8	7	7	6	6	7	8	7	7	7	6	6	7	7	7	8	7	6	6	6	7	8	8	7	6	6	7	7	7	8	7	6
EVENINGS	5	5	7	6	6	6	5	5	6	6	6	6	6	5	5	6	6	6	6	6	5	5	5	6	6	6	6	5	5	5	6	6	7	6	5	5	5	6	6	7	6	5
NIGHTS	3	3	3	3	4	2	2	3	3	4	3	3	2	2	3	3	4	3	3	2	2	3	3	4	3	3	2	2	3	3	4	3	3	2	2	3	3	4	3	3	2	2
TOTALS	14	15	17	16	18	15	13	14	16	17	17	16	15	13	14	16	18	16	16	15	13	14	15	17	16	17	15	13	14	14	17	17	18	15	13	14	15	17	16	18	15	13

Fig. 4-5. Model staff schedule.

and educational needs of the nursing staff and provide commensurate programs to meet those needs. Like the head nurse, they can stagger their hours to meet with the night shift to evaluate ongoing in-service programs or provide new programs.

Note that this schedule does not demonstrate staffing patterns for holidays, vacations, or sick time. It is understandable that fewer staff members would be available during those times, and the unit can be supplemented by a "float pool" from other primary nursing units, if they exist, or by floating personnel from other units. (Also, if this unit is overstaffed and another unit is understaffed, it is conceivable that staff from this unit might be floated.)

THE DISTRIBUTION OF WORK FOR NURSING STAFF

Patient assignments on a primary nursing unit provide continuity of care to patients and are determined by primary and associate nurses and by the needs of the patient which are based on comprehensive assessments. Although the model unit is staffed only with R.N.s, L.V.N.s as primary nurses and the "buddy system" will be discussed in Chapter 5 as an alternative approach to primary nursing.

Patient assignment sheets on a primary nursing unit reflect more than the number of patients assigned to each nurse. They indicate who are primary nurses and who are associate nurses, additional staff assignments, and scheduled in-service activities. Fig. 4-6 is an example of a daily patient assignment sheet and provides the head nurse and staff members easy reference to primary and associate nurses. In addition, this assignment sheet informs the ward clerk, unit manager, or supervisor about who the primary nurses are for physicians, family, or other hospital personnel. It is suggested that student nurses be assigned directly to the staff nurses with whom they will be collaborating. In this way the lines of communication are understandable for the nursing staff.

Assignments of float personnel coming to the unit can be made in a similar way to student nurses and on the basis of their abilities and the needs of the patients. If float personnel are coming to the unit for successive days, it is important that every effort be made to assign them the same patients and the same R.N. to collaborate with to provide continuity and coordination of care.

As demonstrated in Fig. 4-6, staff nurses may not have equal numbers of patients assigned to them. Comprehensive patient assessments reveal that priorities and in depth nursing care for each patient can differ greatly. Nurse A has selected and is assigned only three patients because the problems and needs of those patients will employ the nurse's attention for the entire shift. On the other hand, Nurse C has six patients and is the primary nurse for two patients and is the associate nurse for the remaining four patients. It can be hypothesized that those patients are convalescing or near the end of their hospitalization and require less acute attention and comprehensive planning. In summary, it can be formulated that an individual patient's holistic needs, based on a comprehensive assessment, equal the amount of time needed by a single nurse for planning, coordinating, evaluating, and providing continuity of care to the patient.

P = Primary Nurse   DAILY PATIENT ASSIGNMENT   A = Associate Nurse

UNIT____   DATE____   SHIFT 7:00-3:30   CHARGE NURSE____

NURSE A-RN	NURSE B-RN	NURSE C-RN	NURSE D-RN	NURSE E-RN	NURSE F-RN	NURSE G-RN
P 301 P 305A P B	P 306A P B P 304	P 302 P 303 A 307A A B A C A D	A 308A A B A C A D P 310A P B	P 309A P B A C A D A 314	A 312A A B P 313A P B	P 311A P B A 315
LUNCH:						IN-SERVICE: 1:00-1:30 Dr. Smith "Death & Dying" 1:30-2:00 Pt.-Cent. Conference (Nurse G)
LUNCH:						

Fig. 4-6. Daily patient assignment.

THE ORGANIZATION OF SHIFTS FOR
PATIENT CARE CONTINUITY

On a primary nursing unit, all staff members for each shift listen to the full patient report from the previous shift. In addition to making a report on their assigned patients, staff are encouraged to note the highlights of care given to the remaining patients on the unit. Physicians, families, and other hospital personnel may approach any staff nurse inquiring about specific patients. The staff nurse can provide the necessary information or refer the person seeking information to the appropriate primary nurse.

		Team Nursing	Primary Nursing
A.	Admission Procedure	1. Patients assigned to nurses not busy or by room assingment.	1. Patients selected by a primary nurse based on the nurse's abilities and the patient's needs, indicating the selection in the appropriate areas.
		2. Routine hospital admission form used.	2. The primary nurse initiates an admission interview which includes a nursing history and physical.
		3. Patient is usually followed the rest of the shift by the admitting nurse although that varies, i.e., the team leader might admit and a team member follow the patient.	3. The primary nurse becomes accountable for the patient's care not only for the shift but for the duration of hospitalization.
		4. Head Nurse or team leader initiates physician's orders.	4. The primary nurse communicates admission findings to the head nurse and physician and initiates the physician's orders.
		5. The head nurse co-signs the orders, communicates them to the team leader who communicates them to the team member(s).	5. The primary nurse co-signs physician's orders and provides feedback to the Head Nurse.
		6. The team leader or team member initiates a care plan on the Kardex.	6. The primary nurse initiates a twenty-four hour care plan on the primary nursing care plan and records pertinent observations on the Kardex. This plan of care includes patient participation.

Fig. 4-7. A comparison of team and primary nursing.

	Team Nursing	Primary Nursing
A. continued	7. The team leader is accountable for patient's care after admission for that particular shift.	7. The primary nurse is accountable for the twenty-four hour planning for patient care and includes assessment, evaluation, and communication.
	8. The patient is oriented to the physical structure of the unit.	8. The patient is oriented to the physical structure of the unit, primary nursing and introduced to selected associate nurses.
B. Nursing Assessment	1. Usually by team member-team leader if team member not qualified.	1. Primary Nurse-Associate Nurse, secondarily. (Both may be qualified.)
C. Nursing Tasks	1. Same as B.	1. Same as B.
D. Carrying Out Doctor's Orders, e.g., medications and treatments	1. Usually Team Leader	1. Primary Nurse or Associate Nurse
E. Communication Lines Regarding Patient Care	1. Physician ↓ ↑ ↓ Head Nurse ↓ ↑ ↓ Team Leader ↙ ↙ ↘ ↘ Team Members	1. Communication triangle between Physician, Head Nurse, and Primary Nurse. Physician △ Primary Nurse Head Nurse
F. Accountability for Patient Care	1. Team leader for team-reports to head nurse. 2. Team members for some aspects of patient care depending on their ability. Reports to team leader.	1. Primary Nurse accountable for all aspects of patient care-provides feedback to Head Nurse.
G. Continuity of Care	1. Patients are not assured same nurses. 2. Team usually stable but team leaders may vary.	1. Patients assured same nurses on all three shifts throughout hospitalization. 1. Primary Nurse plans for patient care on a twenty-four hour basis during entire hospitalization; associate nurse follows through on the plan.

Continued.

Fig. 4-7, cont'd. For legend see opposite page.

	Team Nursing	Primary Nursing
H. Patient Assignments	1. Example: Day shift—7 staff, assigned 30 bed unit—2 teams. Head Nurse 2 team members 5 team members Head Nurse Team Leader Team Leader 6 6 6 6 6 Six patients to each team member.	1. Example: Day shift—7 staff assigned 30 bed unit—primary nursing. Head Nurse 7 staff members Head Nurse 3 3 6 6 5 4 3 3-6 patients each staff member.
I. Shift Report	1. Head Nurse and team leader hear and take report for specific teams. 2. Team members hear report from team leaders after shift report—may occur 30-90 minutes after coming on duty. 3. The team leader gives report to the oncoming team leader for the team.	1. All nurses hear and take report directly from the previous shift on all patients. 2. Primary nurses make patient rounds after report and review and plan care for the day. 3. Individual staff members tape report for the oncoming shift on their individual patients.
J. Discharge Planning	1. Head Nurse, team leader, and sometimes team member.	1. Primary nurse with associate nurse follow-through.
K. Quality of Care	1. Continuity of care not consistent. 2. Assignments not consistent. 3. Patient assignments usually greater in number giving nurses time to only provide basic care. 4. Rationale for care and orders communicated through channels—team members rarely receive first-hand communication.	1. Continuity of care insured. 2. Assignment planning consistent. 3. Patient assignments often less, providing nurses more time to plan care and spend time with patients. 4. Communication triangle provides nurse first-hand rationale for care.

Fig. 4-7, cont'd. For legend see p. 58.

After the shift report the primary nurse formulates an organizational plan of patient care for the day, which includes intervention by other hospital personnel and physician's rounds. Patients are familiarized with tests, treatments, teaching, or surgery for that day during the primary nurse's initial patient rounds. The primary nurse plans for time during the shift for patient assessment, evaluating care plans, coordinating care through hospital and community resources, and communicating with the head nurse, associate nurse, and physician.

To understand the organization for primary nursing, it is helpful to compare it to another patient care delivery system such as team nursing, as shown in Fig. 4-7. Fig. 4-7 can be referred to throughout this chapter for specific references to the primary nurse's activities. We are interested in making this comparison not only to show differences in the approaches of patient care modalities but also to specifically state the components of primary nursing.

Inherent in primary nursing is the total care of one patient by one nurse. Primary nurses provide total care to all patients assigned to them. More specifically this includes nursing tasks, such as giving baths, changing linens, taking vital signs, giving medications and treatments, and charting. Staff nurses on a primary nursing unit are accountable for cosigning physician's orders and for validating their accuracy after they are transcribed. Head nurses can also validate the accuracy of transcribed orders and communicate those orders needing immediate attention to the staff nurse. However, staff nurses are encouraged to check physician's orders to discourage obstruction of communication, thereby enchancing safe patient care.

Physicians arriving on a primary nursing unit will ask specifically for the patient's primary nurse, and this information can be made available in several ways. The assignment sheet is one way and has already been discussed. Another source of this information is shown in Fig. 4-8, which is an example of a label that can be utilized on the front of the chart. Primary and associate nurses and their corresponding shifts are stated on the label, thus providing the physician a quick reference, regardless of the time he arrives on the unit. Furthermore, with this labeling system, other hospital personnel can ask for specific nurses.

After the basic nursing care has been given, the afternoon can be spent following through on patient problems, reevaluating and planning for patient needs and care, and reflecting changes on the nursing care plan. Admission interviews, family conferences, and discharge planning can be scheduled for the afternoon. Staff meetings and in-service conferences can be arranged in advance and posted on the assignment sheet so that staff can plan their work to include time to attend.

Although the organization of care has been presented in the traditional time sequence, which is baths in the morning and conferences in the afternoon, it is not essential or even necessarily practical to follow this pattern in primary nursing. It is often more effective and relevant to organize care, when possible, for the comfort and convenience of the patient. For example, a patient who always bathes in the evening at home can be given the preference to bathe in the evening

```
┌─────────────────────────────────────────────┐
│                                             │
│              _____               │
│              PHYSICIAN                       │
│                                             │
│                                             │
│   _____                 │
│   PRIMARY NURSE              SHIFT           │
│                                             │
│                                             │
│   _____                 │
│   ASSOCIATE NURSE            SHIFT           │
│                                             │
│                                             │
│   _____                 │
│   ASSOCIATE NURSE            SHIFT           │
│                                             │
│                                             │
│   _____                 │
│   ASSOCIATE NURSE            SHIFT           │
│                                             │
└─────────────────────────────────────────────┘
```

Fig. 4-8. Primary nursing chart label.

in the hospital. The laborer who has always eaten dinner at 4:30 P.M. every evening for ten years can be given the preference of an early dinner rather than wait for the hospital appointed hour of 6 P.M. Most hospital departments are more than willing to extend individual courtesies to patients if they are notified of patients' desires.

Shift reports on a model unit are taped because taping provides a more efficient and pertinent form of reporting (see discussion in Chapter 5). Primary nurses particularly emphasize and highlight follow through of teaching, specific patient approaches, patient priorities, significant changes, and appropriate planning to provide for the changes. While the evening shift is hearing reports, the day staff completes its charting and continues to answer patient needs. Following the shift report, primary and associate nurses discuss in greater depth specific patient management and together make rounds on the primary nurse's patients to enhance continuity of care.

The evening shift can continue with an organization similar to the day shift and can also organize the shift to meet patient needs on a highly individual basis. Patient assignments continue to be based on needs of the patients and the time it takes to meet those needs and, like the day shift assignments, may not be equally divided among the nurses. Evening nurses also formulate an organizational plan of care for their patients, and this plan includes follow through on patient problems and needs, teaching, family interaction, and physician rounds.

Patients admitted on the evening shift are selected by primary nurses who, in turn, select associate nurses on the other shifts. The accountability of the evening shift primary nurse remains the same as the day shift primary nurse. The evening shift primary nurse, in addition to selecting associate nurses, makes the initial comprehensive patient assessment, initiates a primary nursing care plan, and communicates and coordinates the care plan. The patient is continually evaluated by the primary nurse, who communicates necessary changes in patient status for the duration of the patient's hospitalization. The communication triangle on the evening shift consists of the physician, the primary nurse, and the assistant head nurse. The head nurse continues to receive feedback concerning the patient's management, but the assistant head nurse is an integral part of the triangle on the evening shift.

Assistant head nurses on the evening shift are the clinical and organizational stabilizing forces for the shift. In complementary roles to head nurses, they collaborate with head nurses as resource people, role models, and unit coordinators. They assist the nursing staff to problem solve more effectively and thus to arrive at more independent decision making. Like head nurses, they maintain communication with the staff concerning changes in patient status and assist in determining priorities for patient care.

Although most hospitals employ assistant head nurses or charge nurses on the evening shift to act in a charge nurse capacity, it is not necessarily practical to designate an evening "charge person" on the model unit. The assistant head nurse on this unit can perhaps be more effective working in a horizontal relationship to staff, that is, selecting primary patients and thereby demonstrating the function of role model operationally. The assistant head nurse would have fewer patients to allow enough flexibility to assist other staff members during the evening as problems and/or questions arise.

This milieu can encourage staff members to become more independent in their nursing practice and at the same time give staff a resource person with whom to collaborate. Their individual leadership skills as well as their efficiency can be enhanced by allowing them greater responsibility and recognition for their ability.

It is suggested that the primary nurse role be confined to the day and evening shift. The night shift is often an impractical time to select patients on most hospital units. Sleeping patients, few admissions, and rare family interactions are not conducive to the primary nurse–patient relationship. However, the climate is different on acute care units, and there might be a necessary role for primary nurses on the night shift on these units.

Associate nurses have an important role on the night shift. For example, patients who seem secure and highly cooperative during the day and evening shift may be restless and anxious during the night shift. There can be several reasons for this change, but it is highly important that one nurse, an associate nurse, is present to evaluate the change, determine its reasons, and assist the patient to reach a restful sleep. These changes in patients can often be dismissed by the other shifts because they do not encounter them. The single most important aspect of primary nursing is that the patient's needs are continuously assessed and communicated throughout the twenty-four–hour setting and that no change is too minor to overlook. Primary nursing speaks clearly to the fact that the patient is the center of care and that all nurses on all shifts have the responsibility for the well-being of the patient.

In summary, continuity of patient care is provided when all three shifts work harmoniously, centering their attention on needs of the patients and the best way to meet those needs. In primary nursing, patient-centered care and continuity of care are accomplished by specific nurses designating primary and associate nurse roles on the three shifts. The communication of care through shift report, patient-centered conferences, physician rounds, the communication triangle, and patient rounds by primary and associate nurses ensures patients and their families comprehensive and continous care.

SELECTION OF PRIMARY PATIENTS

A detailed look at the selection of patients by the primary nurse will help to describe more specifically the process of primary nursing. A hypothetical patient situation will be utilized to describe more fully the primary nurse-patient relationship. Included in this discussion will be the nursing history and physical of the patient on admission, the primary nursing care plan, the primary nursing board, and the Kardex care plans.

Patients are selected by primary nurses on the basis of the nurses' abilities and needs of the patients. The questions "What if the nurse is a bad nurse?," "What if the patient doesn't like the nurse?," or "What if the patient is a demanding patient?" have certainly been raised. On a primary nursing unit, nurses must continually ask themselves those same questions and find answers to them. With the help of the head nurse and other advisory personnel, nurses must also continually assess their abilities, performance, and attitudes so that they may develop their limited areas and utilize their abilities to benefit the patient most. "Bad" patients often act out their purported badness to get attention from nurses, that is, to get someone to care about them, using the only mechanism they have available to them at the time, which is being antagonistic, demanding, or sullen.

In primary nursing the selection of patients on admission lets the patient know immediately that someone, the primary nurse, will care about him, not just during the admission procedure but for the duration of the hospitalization. The patient is further informed that other nurses, associate nurses, will take care of him and be responsive to his needs in the primary nurse's absence. As the associate nurses are selected, they are introduced to the patient, who soon after admission comes to know the specific people to depend on. The patient also learns that "his nurses" are knowledgeable about his illness and that they will include his family in planning care and provide teaching to both the patient and family. The patient learns that community agencies and resources can be employed during the hospitalization and after discharge and that the primary nurse will coordinate these efforts. The patient in this setting has little reason to act "bad," and even if this behavior occurs, there will be a nurse advocate to understand and make the necessary changes to encourage the patient's sense of well-being and trust.

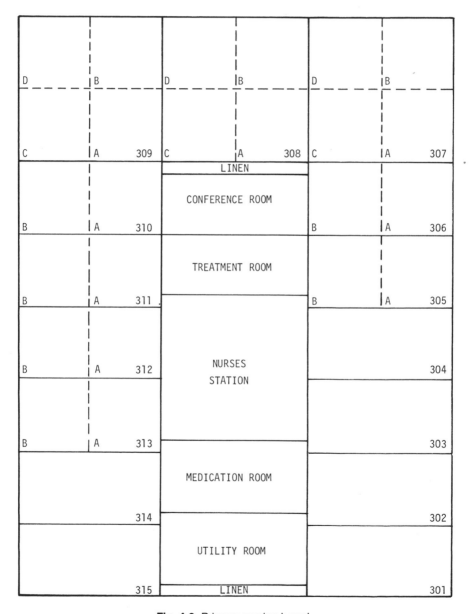

Fig. 4-9. Primary nursing board.

This chapter has discussed in detail the importance of informing staff and hospital personnel about the identity of the primary nurse. Available references to the primary nurse enhance direct communication and allow unit staff members to know what patients have been selected by primary and associate nurses. Fig. 4-9 is an example of a primary nursing board for a hospital medical-surgical unit. This drawing, enlarged and mounted, can serve as a primary nursing board where primary and associate nurses designate their status in the appropriate room numbers. A blackboard can serve the same purpose. The board can be hung at the nurses' station to alert physicians, hospital personnel, and other staff immediately to primary and associate nurses. It can also serve as an excellent reference for the head nurse who, at a glance, can see that all patients have primary nurses and who those primary nurses are. It can also be helpful for nurses returning from days off, illnesses, or vacations to see the possibilities for patient selection.

In the following discussion a hypothetical case is presented, and the activities of the primary nurse are more specifically delineated. The patient is a 45-year-old white woman who enters the hospital with newly diagnosed diabetes mellitus. She is selected by a primary nurse who sees the need for and enjoys diabetic teaching, especially to patients with new diabetics. The primary nurse will plan care and teaching on the basis of an expected ten-day hospitalization.

The admission interview is begun with the patient receiving an explanation of the primary nurse role and the overall philosophy of primary nursing. The patient learns that the primary nurse will be her advocate who will represent her to all personnel involved in her care. The patient learns that she will be introduced to associate nurses who will follow through on the care and teaching planned for the patient and her family.

A comprehensive patient assessment begins on admission to initiate a primary nursing care plan that will be pertinent and reflect the patient's needs and concerns. Thus the nursing interview includes nursing history, a physical examination, a nursing system review, nursing impressions, and discharge planning (Fig. 4-10).

This patient has the typical symptoms of diabetes. It is apparent from her history that the patient has had some problems in the past that might be related to or might complicate the present illness, including weight gain, lack of exercise, and history of hypertension. The patient relates that her husband is Italian and likes spicy Italian foods and wine and that he is not happy about her diagnosis. Her physician has told her that she will be on a strict diabetic diet and that she will take insulin for the rest of her life. She has had two recent hospitalizations and relates that she did not receive the care she had expected. She has managed a dentist's office for twenty years and takes great pride in her ability to handle a difficult job and maintain a home for her husband and two young sons. The patient denies that any family member had diabetes mellitus, and she states frankly that she does not want to have it.

The system review is generally negative, except for the symptoms of diabetes,

A. General Admission Information:

Date _2-28-73_ Time _1⁰⁵ P.m._ Mode _Walking_ Allergies _Penicillin_

TPR _98⁴-88-18_ BP _160/98_ HT _5'2"_ WT _179_ Diet _Regular_

Sleep habits _Fair. Poor when nervous_ CBC: Yes ✓ No_____ Urinalysis: Yes ✓ No_____

Property: Glasses _o_ Contact Lenses _o_ Dentures _o_

        Prosthesis _o_ Ring _Yellow band_ Watch _1- Yellow Timex_

        Money _$10.45_ Other _Radio-Panasonic Transistor_

        Values to Business Office _o_

B. Nursing History:

  1. Chief complaint _"Eating more. Voiding large amt. urine. Thirsty"_
  2. Present Illness (include symptoms) _Above symptoms began three weeks ago - increased over past week._
  3. Past Medical History (especially as it relates to P.I.):
     a. Medical _Weight problems. Hypertension_
     b. Surgical _Abd. hysterectomy 1969   Cholecystectomy 1971._
     c. Allergies _Penicillin, Dust._
     d. Medications _Estrogen. Occas. Lasix_
     e. Traumatic injuries _o_
     f. Orthopedic _o_
  4. Habits:
     a. Smoking _2 packs/day_
     b. Alcohol _Social_
     c. Exercise _Very little_
  5. Social History:
     a. Marital Status: Married ✓ Single____ Divorced____ Widowed____
     b. State of Birth _California_
     c. Education _2 yrs - dental assistant_
     d. Occupation _Office manager for dentist - 20 years_
  6. Family History (circle appropriate illnesses):
    Diabetes (Hypertension) (Cancer) (Heart) Tuberculosis Anemia
    Mental Other_____
  7. Physician's Admitting Diagnosis _Diabetes mellitus_

C. Nursing Review of Symptoms (circle appropriate symptoms):
  1. HEENT: Headaches Hearing loss Vision _20/20_ Diplopia
       Eye pain Eye infections Blurring Epistaxis
       Sinus pain Facial pain Bleeding gums Dentures
       Sore throats Nasal-tracheal pain Other_____
  2. CARDIO-RESPIRATORY: Chest pain (site)_____ _o_
       Chest pain with exertion Dyspnea on exertion
       Nocturnal dyspnea (Edema) (Hypertension) Palpitations
       Known murmur (Cough) (Sputum) Hemoptysis
       Pleuritic pain Diaphoresis Varicosities
    Last Chest X-Ray _1971_ EKG _1972_
    Other_____
  3. GASTROINTESTINAL: (Thirst) Nausea Vomiting Hematemesis
       Heartburn Difficulty swallowing Flatulance
       Abdominal pain Jaundice Diarrhea (Constipation)
       Tarry stools (Hemorrhoids) Hernia Other _Increased appetite_
  4. GENITO-URINARY: Dysuria (Polyuria) Frequency Urgency
       Nocturia Burning Hematuria Stones Incontinence
       Enuresis Retention

Continued.

Fig. 4-10. Primary nursing admission interview.

    a. Female Genital Tract—Menstral History: Age of onset _12 yrs._
       Frequency _o_ Regularity _o_ Duration _o_
       Date last period _1969_ Post menopausal bleeding _o_
       Menopause: Age _o_ Symptoms _____
       Last Serology _1969_
    b. P ♀ 2 G ♀ 2 Ab o
    c. Male Genital Tract—Penile discharge Lesions Testicular pain
       Testicular Swelling Last Serology _____
       Other _____

5. MUSCULO-SKELETAL: Extremity pain Joint pain Back pain
    Muscle pain Neck pain Stiffness Limited motion
    Joint swelling Redness Sprains Deformity
    X-Rays _o_ Other _____

6. NERVOUS: Convulsions Syncope Dizziness Vertigo Tremor
    Ataxia Speech difficulty Limp Paralysis Paresthesias
    Muscle atrophy Muscle tenderness EEG _o_
    Other _____

7. ENDOCRINE: Goiter Tremor Heat or Cold intolerance
    Exophthalmos Voice change (Polydipsia)
    Change in body contour Infertility Other _____

D. Nursing Physical:

1. HEENT
    a. Symmetry _Symmetrical_
    b. Eyes and Pupils _PERL_
    c. Ears _Small amt. wax Eardrum visible_
    d. Mouth and Throat _gums pink. No visible caries. Throat o_
    e. Lymph nodes _None palpable_

2. RESPIRATORY
    a. Depth and Rate _R-18 and deep_
    b. Breath sounds _Clear_
    c. Abnormal sounds _o_
    d. Chest expansion _Good bilaterally_

3. CARDIO-VASCULAR
    a. Blood Pressure (R) _160/98_ (L) _158/94_ Lying _152/92_ Standing _160/96_
    b. Apical pulse and regularity _88 - Regular_
    c. Pedal pulses _Present and strong bilaterally_
    d. Neck vein distention _o_

4. CHEST
    a. Breast mass _None palpable_

5. GASTRO-INTESTINAL
    a. Bowel sounds _Present_
    b. Tenderness or rigidity _o_

6. URINARY
    a. Bladder distention _o_

7. SKELETAL
    a. Arthritic joints _o_
    b. Range of motion _9000_

8. NEURO
    a. Motor paralysis
      1) Facial _o_
      2) Extremities _o_
    b. Sensory (equal or not with pin prick) _Equal_
    c. Equilibrium
      1) Balance _9000_
      2) Finger to nose _OK_
    d. Reflexes (equal or not equal)
      1) Knees _Equal_ 2) Arms _Equal_

Fig. 4-10, cont'd. For legend see p. 67.

E. Nursing Impression: *A well-nourished, obese, intelligent 45 yr. old W ♀ Jc Presenting symptoms of increased appetite, thirst & urine. Evidence of hypertension on admitting. BP status - AP reg - 1sd EKG - 1972. No edema present. Initial urine for S/A 3+ reg. Unable to accept initial diagnosis of diabetes mellitus - related family and cultural problems. Overall prognosis: Fair → good.*

F. Discharge Planning:
   1. Probable Date _10 days_   3/10/73 _____
   2. Destination _Home_ _____
   3. Transportation _Car_   By Whom _Husband_ _____
   4. Agencies and Equipment Involved _diabetic association_ _____
   _____
   5. Diet _diabetic - low cal._ _____
   6. Medications _Insulin_ _____
   7. Person responsible for patient _Mr. Russell Jones_ Phone _276-1777_
   8. Family conference _will plan_ _____
   9. Anticipated problems _some resistance to diabetic regimen._ _____
   10. Home visit _will evaluate._ _____

                              Joan Jones, R.N.
                              Nurse's Signature

Fig. 4-10, cont'd. For legend see p. 67.

hypertension and edema. The patient thinks that the cough and sputum are from smoking, and the physician corroborates this. The physical examination is generally negative. A nursing impression is written that synthesizes all the data gathered during the interview. Discharge planning is begun during the admission interview, using as much available information as possible.

The primary nurse initiates the primary nursing care plan when the admission interview is completed. Including the patient and family in outlining the plan of care and teaching is paramount, especially with this patient. Both the patient and her husband will become aware of the teaching goals and the importance of both of them understanding the disease. This patient's education and occupation indicate to the nurse that the patient will be able to grasp diabetic teaching and that she will be able to become independent in administering insulin injections and will understand the diabetic diet and reactions, that is, shock and coma.

The primary nursing care plan is the most important tool in primary nursing. In addition to calling attention to the specific patient problems, it specifically outlines the nursing action to be taken on a twenty-four–hour basis for the duration of the hospitalization. This care plan (Fig. 4-11) divides the teaching aspects among the three shifts and sets specific goals for when that teaching is to be completed. The nursing care plan written in this manner prevents the nurse from overwhelming the patient and family with too much detail at one time and

Date	Patient Problems	Expected Outcomes	Goals	Nursing Action
3/1	1. Does not accept diag. Neither does husband. 2. Worries about diet restric. at work, home, eating out & entertaining. Husband likes spicy Italian foods.	1. Patient & family to gain understanding of disease process, treatment, and reactions. 2. Full dietary understanding.	3/10	Teaching along with Emotional Support. Include husband in teaching.
				7-3 Shift
			3/2	A. Assess patient & family understanding of disease.
			3/2	B. Contact dietician to begin teaching diet. Show patient sample meals.
			3/3	C. Use visual aids to discuss disease process, reactions.
			3/4	D. Explain and reinforce progress—review visual aids.
			3/5	E. Review diet teaching. Discuss dietetic foods on the market and diabetic cookbooks.
			3/6	F. Review insulin administration. Reinforce.
			3/7	G. Pt self-administers insulin with supervision.
			3/7	H. Evaluate with M.D. & Pt, Diabetic Association, and call them to send literature to hospital.
			3/8	I. Family conference to assess progress and further teaching emphasis.
			3/9	J. Plan for home visit
				Continue to review teaching.
			3/10	K. Home visit
				3-11 Shift
			3/2	A. Reinforce diet teaching.
			3/3	B. Use visual aids for insulin administration.
			3/4	C. Discuss types of insulin and action.
			3/4	D. Practice giving injection and reading syringe.
			3/5	E. Review insulin and injection technique.
			3/6	F. Self-administration of insulin.
			3/7-3/10	G. Continue to review, reinforce, and supervise self administration. Teach husband technique.
				11-7 Shift
			3/2-3/10	Teach urine testing in early A.M. Supervise daily.

Fig. 4-11. Primary nursing care plan, which is concerned with the patient's physical, emotional, and social condition, as well as teaching and other activities.

SAMPLE KARDEX

PATIENT: _____

PRIMARY NURSE: _____

DIAGNOSIS: Diabetus Mellitus

ASSOCIATE NURSES: _____

PATIENT NEEDS	NURSING ACTION
1. Does not accept diagnosis.	1. Teaching a. Disease process b. Medications c. Reactions: coma, shock d. Diet: Include dietician (see chart for specific outline)
2. Support–tries to avoid discussion of diagnosis by talking about her own work environment.	2. Support a. Patient intelligent, professional who needs and can understand explanations for all procedures, medications, etc. b. Bring patient back to subject when teaching. Allow her other times to discuss her work.
3. Family–Husband does not understand or accept diagnosis.	3. Involve husband in teaching aspects. Seek out his questions.

Fig. 4-12. Sample Kardex.

provides a concise account of the amount of teaching involved. As the specific goals are met the primary nurse can either initial, erase, or summarize what has been done. Implicit in a nursing care plan is the continual evaluation of the patient's status, with the necessary changes reflected.

The primary nursing care plan together with the nursing history and physical are placed in the patient's chart in front of the nurse's notes. The nurses notes specifically reflects the patient problem, the nursing action, and results of that action.

It is important that all nursing staff be alerted to the most pertinent patient observations to ensure continuity of care. Fig. 4-12 is an example of a sample Kardex, which the primary nurse can utilize to reflect the highlights of the patient's needs and the nursing action appropriate to meet those needs. The Kardex, which is utilized mainly as an overview and quick reference to patient problems, is a good tool during patient rounds and Kardex review conferences.

The primary nurse can arrange a patient-centered conference for other nursing staff once the care plan is written. A global and holistic representation of the patient's illness is presented, with specific emphasis on the patient's greatest needs. Other staff members are encouraged to contribute their observations and suggestions for nursing action. The primary nurse delegates teaching and other areas of follow through to the other shifts, and the areas delegated are noted in the care plan.

If the patient responds positively to teaching as this patient does, discharge planning can move swiftly. In this case the Diabetic Association can be involved early and asked to send literature to the hospital. The primary nurse can begin planning a home visit to evaluate diet, understanding of medication administration and techniques, family interaction, and acceptance of the illness.

During this patient's hospitalization, the physician and head nurse and patient are informed and involved in assessing and planning for patient care, since they are within the communication triangle. All aspects of patient teaching, nursing care, and patient management are communicated, reevaluated, and validated by means of a dialogue with the people directly accountable for the care of the patient.

At the time of the patient's admission the primary nurse sets the tone for the patient's hospitalization. The patient is given an opportunity to express her fears and apprehensions. The patient is also given the security that one nurse is accountable for and accepts the responsibility for ensuring the patient comprehensive, continuous care in which the patient is the center for planning care. The primary nurse emerges and remains the most knowledgeable nurse during the patient's hospitalization and communicates that knowledge to associate nurses who further ensure the continuity of patient care.

ORGANIZATIONAL FEATURES SPECIFIC TO PRIMARY NURSING

Although much discussion has been devoted in this chapter to various communication modalities, the specific components of those methods have only been generalized. Communication can be most effective if several modalities are utilized. The communication triangle has been discussed in detail as a way of providing direct communication between the three people accountable for patient care management. Kardex review conferences, patient-centered conferences, family conferences, and physician conferences will be discussed as ways of providing communication to the general nursing staff to further enhance continuity of care. In addition, these conferences support the essential ingredient of staff development on a primary nursing unit by providing a teaching and learning milieu for staff that intensifies and/or improves staff performance and knowledge as well as staff interaction.

Kardex review conferences. Kardex review conferences can be planned on a daily basis and should include as many staff members as possible. This form of review and communication provides the staff with an overview of all patients on the unit, in which the highlights of patient needs and nursing action are discussed. The primary or associate nurses can lead the review on their own patients, encouraging staff members to contribute their observations and suggestions.

Kardex review is a helpful communication tool for many reasons. Staff nurses on a primary nursing unit and in the absence of a team leader will usually be asked for patient information by physicians, families, and hospital personnel. After these reviews nursing staff are better able to answer questions and give pertinent information to the person seeking information. Kardex review conferences further stimulate the staff to make and share observations of patients with the primary nurse. Nurses not working closely with certain patients continue to see most patients, even if it is only when passing the breakfast trays. They may note a change in patient behavior only to dismiss it because they assume that "someone knows about it." Kardex review can provide the primary and associate nurses with information that they might be unaware of and stimulate reevaluation of the patient's situation.

Patient-centered conferences. Patient-centered conferences involve an in-depth description of one patient's needs and the nursing action commensurate with those needs, as opposed to Kardex review conferences in which all patients' needs are highlighted. Patient-centered conferences are held as soon as possible after the patient is admitted to establish and communicate the rationale for and approaches to an individual patient's care. The comprehensive, holistic assessment of the patient and the twenty-four–hour primary nursing care plan are shared with the nursing staff.

Patient-centered conferences also describe in depth the medical diagnosis, the medical rationale for care, medications and their use and toxicity, and treatments with specific emphasis for their use with this diagnosis and prognosis. Discharge planning, community intervention, and home visits can be discussed to further enhance patient care coordination.

The primary nursing care plan is reviewed in detail, with staff members ultimately agreeing on specific nursing actions and patient care approaches. Implicit

73

in the discussion are the teaching and supportive measures needed on the other shifts, and therefore nursing staff from all three shifts should try to attend whenever possible. The nursing care plan can also be written during this conference, with all staff participating in an effort to coordinate a cohesive approach to an individual patient. Another alternative when having patient-centered conferences is to have the physician and primary nurse present the conference together. This approach can demonstrate the colleagueship between physician and primary nurse as well as provide a highly stimulating learning experience for staff. The physician can present the diagnosis, rationale, and plan for patient care from a medical viewpoint. The primary nurse can present the diagnosis, rationale, and plan for patient care from the nursing viewpoint.

Documentation of these conferences is routine, and notes can be taken by any staff member present. The in-service coordinator can keep the minutes in the in-service manual, which is available for general staff review.

Family conferences. In-hospital family conferences can be held to aid family members in understanding and accepting the patient's diagnosis, prognosis, and limitations and to provide information concerning hospital and community resources. The hypothetical case previously discussed will serve to illustrate the importance of family conferences.

It is apparent in this patient's situation that the family, particularly the husband, is going to influence greatly the patient's attitude toward accepting her diagnosis. On the primary nursing care plan (Fig. 4-11) the patient and family are assessed immediately concerning their understanding of the diagnosis. The husband is included in all aspects of teaching, and the family's understanding of that teaching is reviewed continuously. Another family conference is scheduled a couple of days prior to discharge to again assess the patient's and husband's progress and to decide what aspects of teaching need to be further highlighted.

The conference with this family would emphasize their style of living after the patient returns home. Diet, medications, and possible reactions are again reviewed, with time allowed for the patient and husband to express questions, doubts, and apprehension or understanding and acceptance. During the final family conference, tentative dates and the rationale for a home visit by the primary nurse can be discussed. The date for the visit can be finalized with the patient.

Family conferences for surgical patients can be held prior to surgery as well as prior to discharge. The family can be given specific information on what to expect after surgery, such as intravenous feeding, coughing and deep breathing, turning, catheterization, and other matters. Family conferences attempt to allay the family's apprehension and at the same time provide suggestions to the family concerning supportive measures for the patient.

Family conferences as a communication modality enhance the family's understanding and support as well as provide the primary nurse an additional patient observation. Associate nurses can be included in or initiate family conferences as a way of further assessing the holistic patient situation.

Physician conferences. The physician on a primary nursing unit is an integral part of the communication triangle and acts as the chief medical resource person for the primary nurse. Accountability for patient care demands that the nurse have more comprehensive knowledge of that care.

Systems review, symptoms, care of patients with specific diagnoses, and outcomes for those diagnoses are some areas that can be reviewed on a regular basis with physicians. Emotional and supportive care needed for specific patients and diagnoses, with subsequent approaches to those patients, can also be included in the discussions.

Nurses can learn individual physician approaches to patients as well as individual physician preferences for care and patient teaching rationales. Similarly, physicians will come to understand and reinforce nurses' abilities for providing care in the patient care setting as well as respect an individual nurse's rationale for planning, problem solving, and decision making.

SUGGESTED READINGS

A quality control plan for nursing services, Los Angeles, 1965, Committee for Administrative Services in Hospitals.

Bower, F. L.: The process of planning nursing care, St. Louis, 1972, The C. V. Mosby Co.

Brink, P. J.: Natural triad in health care, American Journal of Nursing **72:**897-900, 1972.

Cornell, S. H., and Brush F.: Systems approach to nursing care plans, American Journal of Nursing **71:**1376-1378, 1971.

Edgecumbe, R. H.: The CASH approach to hospital management engineering, Hospitals **39:**70-74, March, 1965.

Lambertson, E.: Nursing care plans should reflect present and future patient needs, Modern Hospital **103:**128, Oct., 1964.

Leimo, A.: Planning patient centered care, American Journal of Nursing, 52, March, 1952.

Mayers, M. G.: A systematic approach to the nursing care plan, New York, 1972, Appleton-Century-Crofts.

Price, E. M.: Staffing for patient care, New York, 1971, Springer Publishing Co., Inc.

Prior, J. A., and Silberstein, J. S.: Physical diagnosis, St. Louis, 1973, The C. V. Mosby Co.

chapter 5

ORGANIZATIONAL FEATURES THAT ENHANCE PRIMARY NURSING

Nursing leaders are always seeking new ways to augment staff efficiency. At the same time they are looking for ways to improve comprehensive care to patients. Although the process of primary nursing can ensure comprehensive and individualized care to a single patient, additional tools can be employed to further enhance continuity, communication, coordination, and organization of patient-centered care to primary patients.

Frequently, tools have to be developed to meet the specific requirements of a new system. In primary nursing, nurses become more independent and thus need better instruments for evaluation and education if they are to enhance their performance and deliver high-quality patient care.

Some of these tools have already been discussed in Chapter 4. In this chapter specific attention will be given to (1) tools that enhance coordination and continuity of patient care, (2) complementary roles in primary nursing not yet discussed, and (3) special tools that promote patients' involvement in their own care.

TOOLS THAT ENHANCE COORDINATION AND CONTINUITY

Improved staff coordination facilitates patient safety, comprehensive patient-centered care, and continuity of patient care. At the same time, patient care becomes more individualized by nurses identifying and communicating the specific information pertinent to each patient's care for the duration of the patient's hospitalization.

In primary nursing, staff coordination and continuity of patient care can be facilitated by employing organizational features that provide nurses the time and tools to achieve their objectives for patient care. Similarly, staff development is facilitated by allowing staff nurses the opportunities they need to achieve their individual objectives for personal and professional development. Taped shift reports, the ten-hour day/four-day week home visits, and shift rotation are some ways that improve staff coordination, continuity of patient care, and staff development.

Taped shift reports. Taping shift reports is one way that staff can be alerted to all patient needs. It also can increase efficiency by eliminating the distractions that often occur during report. With the primary nursing system, nurses know much about a few patients and generally little about many patients. For overall patient safety, it is wise to keep staff at least partially informed about other patients on the unit, in addition to their primary patients. Furthermore, taped reports enhance the pertinence of patient information communicated to the oncoming shift.

For taping reports each nursing unit can establish its own guidelines for communicating the more relevant aspects of patient care, teaching, and follow through. A sample guideline follows:

1. Nurses are to speak slowly and clearly so that notes can be taken by the oncoming shift.
2. Nurses are to have their report well organized before beginning to tape.
3. Nurses are to introduce themselves at the beginning of the tape before giving the patient report.
4. The patient's name, diagnosis, physician, and room number are to be stated.
5. Significant events and new orders from the previous shift are to be conveyed.
6. A brief account of the patient's condition on the present shift, including new orders, is to be given. If further discussion is necessary, it should be indicated that a more detailed discussion will take place with the patient's nurse after report.
7. Primary nurses are to communicate any changes in patient teaching or follow through during the report. Again, detailed discussions with associate nurses can be held after the report.
8. The blood pressure range, elevated temperatures, intravenous feedings, and intake and output are to be recorded if appropriate.
9. The number of times that the patient was medicated for pain and the last time that the medication was given are to be stated.
10. The nurse who is taping is to alert the charge nurse after the report about any problem areas.

In reports about preoperative patients, nurses are to state that the chart is in order for surgery or list incomplete areas, such as the laboratory work, the patient's history, and/or the physical examination. Preoperative teaching including areas of instruction and how teaching is received by the patient and family is to be stated, as well as surgery time and medications.

For fresh postoperative patients, nurses report the time that the patient arrived from the recovery room, his general condition, vital signs, dressings, voiding, diet tolerance, productive or unproductive cough, and patency of tubes such as Foley, nasogastric, and chest tubes. In addition, the nurse includes the patient's and family's emotional status and their understanding of the surgery and treatment measures such as subsequent dressings and tubes. The nurse communicates that appropriate steps were taken to enhance their understanding and acceptance.

A nursing unit might decide to implement taped reports for several reasons. Taping shift reports, as opposed to verbal reporting, economizes time because nurses must be much better organized to tape the report and relay all necessary information concerning a patient's care. Pertinent patient information is communicated to the oncoming shift without interruption or "small talk" among staff members during report. During taped report the entire staff listens to and takes notes on every patient as well as their primary patients. Time for additional problem solving and discussion of problem areas is provided after report.

The ten-hour day/four-day week. As staff nurses become familiar with primary nursing, one of the most frequent questions asked is: "How will I find time to do all those things for my patients when I barely get my work done now?" One alternative, flexibility within the eight-hour day, was discussed in Chapter 4. Another alternative, the ten-hour day, provides nurses ample time for assessing patients, planning primary nursing care, and fostering continuity and coordination of patient care.

Many hospitals across the country are already employing the ten-hour day, and still others are considering its implementation. The impact that this change has on patient care and staff nurses' attitudes has often been exciting as well as cost-effective. The advantages to the patients come from nurses having enough time to plan their care. The advantages to the staff nurse are the necessary time to fulfill the role of primary nurse and having every other weekend off with several sequential days off. The advantage to the hospital is fewer sick hours to pay, since nurses are getting enough time off to rest, to get refreshed and remotivated, and to meet their own personal responsibilities. The hospital also benefits from fewer overtime hours of nurses, since nurses have the time to complete their basic care as well as to highlight patient care within the ten-hour day.

Scheduling methods for the ten-hour day vary from hospital to hospital, depending on each hospital's needs, limitations, and unique circumstances. Fig. 5-1 is an example of a ten-hour schedule with a full complement of twenty-three staff members and demonstrates the staffing on all three shifts. Although the number of staff on each shift on a ten-hour schedule is less than that on an eight-hour schedule, it is important to remember that during the overlap times two shifts are on duty. Note also that one night nurse is working an eight-hour shift. This is to demonstrate that when staffing is short or during vacations, changing some staff to an eight-hour schedule may sometimes be necessary to provide adequate coverage for a shift.

Some hospitals schedule two ten-hour shifts and one four-hour shift, the latter consisting of part-time employees. Other hospitals utilize the ten-hour shift for all three shifts, with a two-hour overlap for each shift. It is this type of scheduling that will be discussed.

Although the ten-hour day in some cases may limit the number of days in sequence that staff are on duty, it does provide the overlap time that nurses need to do the things that ensure individualized patient care.

The ten-hour day for all three shifts can be organized in the following manner:

DAYS: 7:00 A.M. to   5:30 P.M.
EVENINGS: 1:00 P.M. to 11:30 P.M.
NIGHTS: 11:00 P.M. to   9:30 A.M.

	MARCH													
DAYS	S	M	T	W	Th	F	S	S	M	T	W	Th	F	S
	1	2	3	4	5	6	7	8	9	10	11	12	13	14
1A Head Nurse	X				X	X						X	X	X
1B In-Serv. Coord.		X	X				X	X	X	X				
1C		X				X	X	X	X	X				
1D	X	X	X							X	X			X
1E		X				X	X	X	X				X	
1F	X			X	X							X	X	X
1G			X	X			X	X	X	X				
1H	X				X	X						X	X	X
1I		X	X				X	X	X		X			
1J	X			X	X						X		X	X
1K				X		X	X	X			X	X		
EVENINGS														
2A Assist. H.N.		X	X				X	X	X	X				
2B	X	X		X							X	X		X
2C					X	X	X	X				X	X	
2D	X	X	X							X	X			X
2E				X		X	X	X	X	X				
2F	X				X	X					X		X	X
2G			X	X			X	X	X				X	
2H	X				X	X						X	X	X
NIGHTS														
3A					X	X	X	X			X	X		
3B	X	X		X								X	X	X
3C			X			X	X	X	X	X				
3D 8-hr. Rotation	X				X								X	X
DAYS	5	5	6	6	6	5	4	4	5	6	6	6	5	5
EVENINGS	4	5	5	5	5	4	4	4	5	5	5	5	4	4
NIGHTS	2	3	3	3	2	2	2	2	3	3	3	2	2	2
TOTAL	11	13	14	14	13	11	10	10	13	14	14	13	11	11

DAYS	S	M	T	W	Th	F	S	S	M	T	W	Th	F	S
	15	16	17	18	19	20	21	22	23	24	25	26	27	28
1A Head Nurse	X				X	X						X	X	X
1B In-Serv. Coord.		X	X				X	X	X	X				
1C		X				X	X	X	X			X		
1D	X	X	X							X	X			X
1E		X	X				X	X	X				X	
1F	X			X	X						X		X	X
1G			X	X			X	X	X	X				
1H	X			X	X							X	X	X
1I					X	X	X	X			X	X		
1J	X	X				X					X		X	X
1K				X		X	X	X	X	X				
EVENINGS														
2A Assist. H.N.		X	X				X	X	X	X				
2B	X	X	X						X				X	X
2C					X	X	X	X				X	X	
2D	X	X				X					X		X	X
2E		X				X	X	X			X	X		
2F	X			X	X					X			X	X
2G			X	X			X	X	X	X				
2H	X			X	X						X	X		X
NIGHTS														
3A					X	X	X	X	X	X				
3B	X	X		X								X	X	X
3C			X			X	X	X			X	X		
3D 8-hr. Rotation	X				X								X	X
DAYS	5	5	6	6	6	5	4	4	5	6	6	6	5	5
EVENINGS	4	4	5	5	5	5	4	4	5	5	5	5	4	4
NIGHTS	2	3	3	3	2	2	2	2	3	3	3	2	2	2
TOTAL	11	12	14	14	13	12	10	10	13	14	14	13	11	11

				APRIL										
DAYS	S	M	T	W	Th	F	S	S	M	T	W	Th	F	S
	29	30	31	1	2	3	4	5	6	7	8	9	10	11
1A Head Nurse	X				X	X						X	X	X
1B In-Serv. Coord.		X	X				X	X	X	X				
1C		X				X	X	X	X					
1D	X	X	X							X	X			X
1E					X	X	X	X	X				X	
1F	X			X	X							X	X	X
1G		X				X	X	X	X	X				
1H	X			X	X						X		X	X
1I				X		X	X	X			X	X		
1J	X	X	X						X	X				X
1K			X	X			X	X			X	X		
EVENINGS														
2A Assist. H.N.		X	X				X	X	X	X				
2B	X		X	X						X	X			X
2C					X	X	X	X			X	X		
2D	X	X	X						X				X	X
2E				X	X		X	X	X				X	
2F	X	X				X				X	X			X
2G				X		X	X	X				X	X	
2H	X				X	X						X	X	X
NIGHTS														
3A		X				X	X	X	X		X			
3B	X	X		X						X			X	X
3C					X	X	X	X	X			X		
3D 8-hr. Rotation	X				X								X	X
DAYS	5	5	6	6	6	5	4	4	5	6	6	6	4	5
EVENINGS	4	5	5	5	5	4	4	4	5	5	5	5	4	4
NIGHTS	2	3	3	3	2	2	2	2	2	3	3	3	2	2
TOTAL	11	13	14	14	13	11	10	10	12	14	14	14	10	11

Fig. 5-1. Sample ten-hour day/four-day week schedule.

SHIFT	TIME	Eight-hour Day	SHIFT	TIME	Ten-hour Day
7:00 A.M.-3:30 P.M.	7:00-7:30	Shift Report	7:00 A.M.-5:30 P.M.	7:00-7:30	Shift Report
	7:30-11:30	AM Care—Baths, Medications, Treatments, Doctor Rounds, Procedures, Charting		7:30-11:30	AM Care—Baths, Medications, Treatments, Doctor Rounds, Procedures, Charting
	11:30-1:00	Lunch for Patients and Staff		11:30-1:00	Lunch for Patients & Staff
	1:00-1:30	Staff Conference, In-service, etc.		1:00-1:30	Staff Conference, In-service, etc.
	1:30-2:30	Afternoon treatments, Medications, Procedures, Receive Surgical Pts.		1:30-2:30	Afternoon treatments, Medications, Procedures, Receive Surgical Patients
	2:30-3:00	Complete Charting		2:30-3:00	Complete Charting
	3:00-3:30	Report		3:00-3:30	Report
				3:30-5:30	In-service, Patient-centered Conferences, Home Visits, Staff and Unit Projects, Select and Interview Patients, Patient teaching, Care Plans, Work with PMs if necessary, Meet with Primary & Associate Nurses
3:00 P.M.-11:30 P.M.			1:00 P.M.-11:30 P.M.	1:00-3:00	In-service, Patient-centered Conference, Home Visits, Staff and Unit Projects, Interviews, Patient Teaching, Care Plans, Meet with Primary and Associate Nurses, Select Patients
	3:00-3:30	Report		3:00-3:30	Report
	3:30-5:00	Medications, Treatments, Receive Surgical Pts.		3:30-5:00	Medications, Treatments, Receive Surgical Patients

Eight-hour day		Ten-hour day	
		1:00 P.M.– 11:30 P.M.	
5:00–6:30	Staff and Patient Dinner	5:00–6:30	Staff and Patient Dinner
6:00–7:30	Staff Conference	6:00–7:30	Staff Conference
7:00–10:00	Medications, Treatments, Doctor Rounds, Evening Care, Charting, Visiting Hours	7:00–10:00	Medications, Treatments, Doctor Rounds, Evening Care, Charting, Visiting Hours
10:00–11:00	Evening Medications, Complete Charting	10:00–11:00	Evening Medications, Complete Charting
11:00–11:30	Report	11:00–11:30	Report
11:00 P.M.– 7:30 A.M.		11:00 P.M.– 9:30 A.M.	
11:00	Shift Report	11:00	Shift Report
11:30–7:00	Paper Work, Patient Care, Doctor Rounds, Ordering Supplies, Medications, Treatments, Charting, IVs	11:30–7:00	Paper Work, Patient Care, Doctor Rounds, Ordering Supplies, Medications, Treatments, Charting, IVs
7:00–7:30	Report	7:00–7:30	Report
		7:30–9:30	In-service, Patient-centered Conferences, Home Visits, Staff and Unit Projects, Interviews, Patient Teaching, Care Plans, Work with Day Nurses if necessary, Meet with Primary and Associate Nurses

Fig. 5-2. A comparison of nursing activity on the eight-hour and ten-hour day.

The two-hour overlap time is as follows:

DAYS: 3:30 P.M. to   5:30 P.M.
EVENINGS: 1:00 P.M. to   3:00 P.M.
NIGHTS: 7:30 A.M. to   9:30 A.M.

During the ten-hour day, patient care responsibilities can be maintained during the eight-hour shift (such as 7 A.M. to 3:30 P.M.), and the organization of work can be the same as in the traditional eight-hour shift. This type of organization of work allows "float" personnel to come to the unit and fit into the work routine as it appears on every hospital unit. This form of organization also provides the primary nurse with two hours of structured time to devote to the more comprehensive aspects of patient care.

However, redistribution of work can occur within the ten-hour day. For example, bed baths can be done on other shifts to accomodate individual patient needs or desires. Teaching needs of the patient can be met on a more individualized basis for the patient.

The two-hour overlap is the most exciting aspect of the ten-hour day; it is a time when the primary nurse and the patient benefit a great deal. During this time, patient assessments, primary nursing care plans, in-service programs, and unit and individual nursing projects can be planned, implemented, and communicated to patients and other staff members.

It is most important that hospitals recognize this overlap as direct patient care hours. During the overlap, nurses have the opportunity to concentrate on the preventive, holistic, and individualistic needs of patients. Fig. 5-2 demonstrates that the eight-hour day often keeps nurses busy just providing basic nursing care and is just as often task oriented. The ten-hour day in which a two-hour overlap is scheduled for each shift provides nursing hours that are patient-centered.

Communication within the ten-hour day is enhanced because each shift has for four and one-half hour the full complement of two shifts; for eample, from 1 to 5:30 P.M., both the day and evening shift are present. Although the overlap can be utilized by each shift in its own way, it is also possible to incorporate the two shifts for the purposes of admitting patients, following through on patient problems, or assisting the other shift when necessary. Primary nurses and associate nurses can take advantage of this time to communicate and evaluate their plans and assessments of a given patient.

Nurses working the 7 to 5:30 shift, after finishing the basic patient care between 7 and 3:30, can utilize the overlap period in several ways. These include unit in-service programs, patient admission interviews, patient-centered conferences, home visits, and Kardex conferences as well as utilization of hospital and community resources. The overlap time is also a period during which nurses can simply sit and talk with an individual patient, giving him the opportunity to comment on, evaluate, and suggest different ways of meeting his own needs.

The ten-hour day not only fosters a more holistic approach but also provides nurses with the time to communicate about patient care. In addition, nurses have the time to promote and take advantage of educational opportunities that will further enhance their individual abilities and development, thus enabling them to provide more comprehensive patient care.

Home visits. Primary nurses are not only accountable for the twenty-four–hour care given to individual patients for the duration of their hospitalization but also evaluate each patient for a home visit. The primary nurse is the patient's advocate and is also the liaison for the patient between the hospital and the community: that is, the primary nurse plans with the patient and his family continued aid from community resources and makes these resources available to them.

All patients are evaluated for a home visit by the primary nurse, even though some patients may not want a home visit. Although specific reasons for home visits may vary for individual patients, the following objectives of home visits apply to all patients:

1. To promote and provide continuity of care to patients and their families that extends beyond the patients' immediate hospitalization and that enhances each patient's return to his life-style in the community
2. To evaluate the acceptance and understanding of a particular illness and its limitations by patients and their families after they have returned to the community
3. To plan with patients and their families about the use of community resources, which can further enhance the patient's recovery, as well as highlight the preventive aspects of illness
4. To provide communication to the physician and associate nurse concerning patients with a particular illness and their adaptability in the community, thus fostering greater awareness of patients' present and future needs during hospitalization
5. To collaborate with personnel from other health disciplines such as a physical therapist or occupational therapist for comprehension and continuity of care to prevent redundancy in care

One home visit may be all that is necessary for some patients, whereas others may require two or even three home visits. Again, patients are evaluated on an individual basis, and home visits are arranged between the primary nurse and the patient and his family, based on the needs of the patient. It is suggested that home visits be agreed on and scheduled prior to the patient's discharge. Telephone contact can be maintained both before and after home visits. The primary nurse will have to plan for the home visit after evaluating her responsibilities on the unit. If a patient requires several home visits, the primary nurse and the physician can contact community public health agencies to provide the appropriate services to patients.

Primary nurses make home visits to evaluate the patient's status and needs and to contact appropriate agencies as needed. Primary nurses would not necessarily treat the patient in his home and would probably not be covered by the hospital if they did so. Fig. 5-3 is an example of a home visit evaluation form that can be utilized by primary nurses making home visits, with a duplicate going to the patient's physician. This form includes a summary of the patient's history and

Patient's Name_____

Address_____Phone_____

Age_____Marital Status_____Religion_____

Family members_____

Physician_____Address_____Phone_____

Brief Medical History:

Pertinent Past Diagnoses_____

_____

Hospitalizations_____

Community Agencies Involved with Patient's Care_____

_____

Present Patient Status:

Reason for Home Visit_____

Patient's Needs_____

_____

Family Needs_____

Environmental Needs_____

A   Socio-cultural Setting_____

Health-educational Needs_____

Home Visits:

1.   Summary of Visit_____

_____

_____

_____

_____

_____

_____

_____

_____

_____

_____

Follow-up Objectives_____

How Met_____

Visiting Nurse_____Date_____

cc to Dr._____

Fig. 5-3. Home visit evaluation forms. **A,** Home visit. **B,** Follow-up home visit.

present illness and evaluates the present patient environment and the patient's needs in the environment. A summary of the visit is recorded, and follow-up objectives and how these objectives are met are noted. This form allows for three home visits, although three visits are not expected if they are not necessary.

Patient's Name_____

Address_____Phone_____

Reason for Home Visit_____

Physician_____Phone_____

2. Summary of Visit_____
_____
_____
_____
_____
_____
_____
_____
_____

Follow-up Objectives_____
How Met_____
Visiting Nurse_____Date_____

B

3. Summary of Visit_____
_____
_____
_____
_____
_____
_____
_____
_____

Follow-up Objectives_____
How Met_____
Visiting Nurse_____Date_____

cc to Dr._____

Fig. 5-3, cont'd. For legend see opposite page.

Shift rotation. Many hospitals hire nurses for permanent day, evening, and night shifts, with rotation to the other two shifts as the need arises. Although a good deal of support is given to stabilizing nurses and shifts by keeping them on permanent shifts, there are many disadvantages to this form of stabilizing. Nurses consistently working one shift view the needs of the patient and the needs of the unit from only one perspective. Their perceptions can often be distorted. This type of shift assignment can often result in nursing personnel demonstrating

85

loyalty to one shift and to one group of nurses but criticizing other shifts and nurses on those shifts.

Shift rotation provides primary and associate nurses the twenty-four–hour perspective needed to plan and evaluate the twenty-four–hour care for an individual patient. It has been stated that a holistic and comprehensive approach to patients is implicit in primary nursing. Because patients spend twenty-four hours a day and not eight hours a day in the hospital, nurses are better able to grasp the more global aspects of patient care by making direct patient assessments on all three shifts and incorporating that perspective into a nursing care plan.

New employees and, all too often, newly graduated nurses are hired for either permanent evenings or nights, and they are not usually ready or willing to work in an unfamiliar environment with sometimes fewer resources and often greater responsibility. Nurses on a unit with shift rotation can be oriented gradually to all three shifts and, more importantly, can work the day shift until they and their head nurse agree that they are ready to relate to another shift.

Individual nurse development can be enhanced by shift rotation, since different and often greater responsibilities are assumed by nurses working different shifts. In addition to assessing patients' needs from different perspectives, nurses also have the opportunity to take advantage of resources, physician communication, and hospital and community interrelation that might be less readily available on their present shift. Finally, nurses see the operational aspects of a nursing unit in a total perspective and can make suggestions and changes that are necessary and relevant for the unit, staff, and patients.

It is suggested that shift rotation occur with full staff participation for three- to six-week periods. Nurses rotating for one week to the night shift often resist the rotation and, when it occurs, simply "put in their time." This attitude does not lend itself to positive change forces and is demoralizing for the staff who have been assigned to work the shift permanently. A regular rotational pattern with definitive criteria can enhance the colleagueship among nurses that is so vital for working well together on a twenty-four–hour basis in a way that highlights patient care and unit objectives.

COMPLEMENTARY ROLES IN PRIMARY NURSING

Complementary roles can be developed that offer primary and associate nurses resources and tools specific to primary nursing and that enhance staff development and comprehensive patient care. These roles are the unit in-service coordinator, the primary nurse coordinator, the on-call primary nurse, and the buddy to the primary nurse. The traditional nursing leadership roles are examined in Chapter 6, and changes within these roles are suggested to enhance primary nursing.

Unit in-service coordinator. All hospitals (hopefully) have some in-service or ongoing educational programs for the nursing staff. Some hospitals have highly sophisticated in-service departments that offer the staff a variety of programs covering a wide range of disciplines. One pattern is to have an in-service director who delegates the responsibility for unit in-service programs to the head nurse or assistant head nurse. Other hospitals employ staff development coordinators who provide in-service activities to one or more nursing units. Clinical specialists can and often do perform the same service to several units.

Missing from even the most sophisticated in-service departments is one person from each unit who is responsible for evaluating, planning, and implementing in-service conferences that meet the specific needs of each nursing unit and its respective staff. The head nurse's and assistant head nurse's responsibilities are highly global and multifocal. When they have the additional responsibility of providing in-service activities, the in-service programs often become haphazard. This is not necessarily the result of their inability but more often the result of their already existing enormous responsibility of operating a nursing unit on a twenty-four–hour basis.

The unit in-service coordinator role is particularly relevant for a primary nursing unit. Primary and associate nurses need unit in-service programs on a twenty-four–hour basis that will enhance their individual and independent clinical and leadership development. They need to be involved in determining the scope and types of in-service programs as well as to participate in leading and presenting them. They need a coordinator who will work with them and be aware of their special needs and problems to provide both the education and experience that will promote an optimum environment for staff development.

The unit in-service coordinator can maintain the twenty-four–hour unit in-service program as well as the in-service program specific to each shift by rotating shifts and by staggering hours. In this way the coordinator can directly evaluate and affect the quantity and quality of in-service activities needed by staff members on all three shifts. The coordinator can post unit in-service program schedules a month in advance for staff and can incorporate hospital in-service activities into the schedule, thereby coordinating unit and hospital in-service plans with the hospital in-service director.

All in-service conferences held by the staff, physicians, and other personnel can be recorded by nurses attending the conferences, with the minutes maintained by the in-service coordinator in an in-service manual. This manual then is available to staff who are unable to attend the conferences and is a good reference for staff wishing to review a particular program.

The unit in-service coordinator, like the assistant head nurse, can assume the role of primary and associate nurse. In this way the coordinator can be an excellent role model for staff by demonstrating actual ability as well as being a resource person.

Primary nursing coordinator. The role of primary nursing coordinator might be developed by a hospital when primary nursing is implemented on two or more units. The chief focuses for the primary nursing coordinator are educating the nursing staff about primary nursing, supervising the actual implementation process of primary nursing, evaluating primary nursing after implementation, and providing and suggesting new tools relevant to primary nursing.

The primary nursing coordinator can be contacted as nursing units are considered for conversion to primary nursing. The coordinator meets first with the head nurse on that unit and assesses the overall educational needs of the staff, unit problems that might obstruct the implementation process, and unit successes that can be promoted and incorporated to further enhance primary nursing. The coordinator views each unit in an individual way and, without compromising the objectives of primary nursing, assists the nursing staff to incorporate primary nursing in terms of its own needs and goals.

Education of the nursing staff involves all three shifts, and the coordinator must have flexibility of hours to allow for this education. Education for the staff includes delineation of primary and associate nurse roles, physician–primary nurse communication, primary nursing care plans, staff development, interview techniques, the buddy role, and comprehensive patient-centered care. The nursing staff on these units can be informed of evaluation tools for primary nursing as well as tools that enhance primary nursing such as nursing audits. Discussion is focused on the horizontal hierarchy within primary nursing and its inherent lines of communication. New roles such as the unit in-service coordinator can be discussed as a possibility for the unit.

Once the nursing staff is informed about and motivated by the theory of primary nursing, an outline for implementation can be delineated with the staff (see Chapter 6). The primary nursing coordinator, who supervises the actual implementation, can evaluate the rate of progress and ensure that the staff are progressing at a pace that produces positive results.

The primary nursing coordinator role complements the head nurse role, and the coordinator, like the supervisor, advises and recommends to the head nurse but does not have authority over the head nurse. Specifically, the coordinator can assist the head nurse by helping staff nurses align their abilities as primary and associate nurses with the needs of patients. Staff consultations can occur between the coordinator and the primary nurse concerning primary nursing care plans and patient assessments. The primary nursing coordinator and the in-service coordinator can collaborate to provide the necessary tools for enhancement of primary nursing.

After a unit has successfully implemented primary nursing, the primary nursing coordinator becomes less active on the unit. His or her emphasis shifts to the next unit preparing for implementation of primary nursing. After full hospital implementation, the coordinator becomes the chief resource person for primary nursing throughout the hospital. Keeping abreast of and incorporating new trends in nursing, including primary nursing, is now the focus of the coordinator's attention. The coordinator continues to collaborate with head nurses, unit in-service coordinators, supervisors, in-service directors, and the director of nursing to promote a hospital environment that fosters primary nursing and staff development.

The "on-call" primary nurse. Not only is it highly possible, but it is also highly probable that the primary nurse role will be greatly expanded in the future to include the "on-call" primary nurse. Patients might look forward to receiving a telephone call from primary nurses prior to admission to the hospital. Patients might even meet their primary nurses before entering the hospital. Admission interviews might be conducted on an outpatient basis, with a care plan ready when the patient enters the hospital.

As patients are transferred to different units, for example, the intensive care unit (I.C.U.) to a medical-surgical unit, their care might be followed through on the new unit by their I.C.U. primary nurse. At the least the I.C.U. primary nurse might serve in a continuing consultant role to the primary nurse on the medical-surgical unit.

Some primary nurses will see patients on an outpatient basis, admit them, and become their primary nurses, follow them through the hospitalization, and make home visits. Pediatrics is certainly one area that would benefit from an expanded primary nurse role.

The role of "on-call" primary nurses will be further examined by presenting a hypothetical situation in which "on-call" primary nurses are working on an obstetrical unit (another area that could benefit greatly from an expanded primary nurse role). The basic premise for the "on-call" role is complete nurse mobility and autonomy, which affords the primary nurse the time and flexibility of hours to completely coordinate with the physician the patient's care from onset of pregnancy through follow-up during the postpartum period.

Primary nurses can select obstetrical patients in several ways. Physicians who understand and support the objectives of a primary nursing unit can refer patients who need to be followed through. The primary nurse can then contact the physician's nurse, learn the next appointment date, and, together with the physician, see the patient in the physician's office. Staff nurses presenting parent classes can select patients at an early class and follow through on these patients from then on.

The primary nurse can plan to see the patient each office visit; however, it is understandable that the needs of the nurse's newly hospitalized patients may conflict, thus modifying the nurse's prenatal involvement. The patient can call the nurse and relate specific details of the appointment missed by the primary nurse as the patient-primary nurse relationship builds. The primary nurse-physician communication focuses on the teaching needs of the patient and her family, community intervention, and child care.

As the patient's delivery date nears, the primary nurse, like the physician, goes on call for the delivery. The primary nurse is called either by the expectant mother, her husband, or a staff member when the patient is leaving for or has entered the hospital.

The primary nurse stays with the patient and her husband throughout labor. The delivery room nurse can do the actual timing of contractions and other functions of labor nurses or may delegate these functions to the primary nurse. Most important is that the primary nurse assumes a role during labor and delivery that is beneficial to the expectant mother. The primary nurse accompanies the patient to the delivery room and again assumes a supportive role, such as assisting the physician with delivery, staying with the husband, or staying with the new mother. After delivery the primary nurse remains with the new mother until she is comfortable and settled in her room.

From this point on, the primary nurse continues in the role of hospital primary nurse, that is, planning, implementing, and evaluating the twenty-four–hour care for the new mother for the duration of her hospitalization. The primary nurse on this unit further assumes accountability for coordinating the needs of the mother and the new baby, for child care teaching, and for following through.

The new mother, like all primary patients, is evaluated for a home visit. The procedure for making home visits, which includes utilizing the home visit form and sending a copy to the physician, can be the same as with other primary patients. An obstetrical department might want to expand this form to collect data specific to the unit.

An expanded primary nurse role has many advantages for the new mother, especially if this is the first child. All the mother's questions, fears, and apprehensions are answered and alleviated from the time that pregnancy is confirmed. Her life-style with a new baby is discussed long before her actual delivery date. Most importantly, she is followed through for the duration of her pregnancy and hospitalization by one nurse, a primary nurse, who helps to make the entire experience a highly comfortable, educational, and growth-producing experience for the new mother.

At present, schools of nursing approach the teaching of obstetrics in this way; that is, they allow students to follow through on patients during pregnancy and while hospitalized before and after delivery. The students often refer to their patients as "my mother" or "my newborn," just as the mother refers to the student as "my nurse." Why this experience is confined to the student nursing educational process is certainly a question that needs to be raised by staff nurses presently working in obstetrics.

The buddy system. As mentioned previously, agencies are devoting much thought and discussion to the question: "What levels of staff—registered nurses (R.N.s), licensed vocational nurses (L.V.N.s), or nurses' aides (N.A.s)—should participate in the primary nurse role? Some hospitals employ only R.N.s for the role. Others employ L.V.N.s and N.A.s, but only L.V.N.s are primary nurses, not N.A.s. If auxiliary personnel are to be incorporated into the primary nursing system, a modified system is necessary. First, L.V.N.s must select patients according to the needs of the patients and the abilities of the nurse. The "buddy system" is one way of validating and checking out the performance of the L.V.N. and the quality of care received by each patient.

A primary nurse, whether an R.N. or L.V.N., or an associate nurse would be expected to relate to the buddy in the following ways:

1. Take full patient report
2. Know the capabilities and limitations of assigned buddies
3. Make complete patient rounds on buddy's patients in addition to rounds on assigned patients

4. Discuss selection of primary and associate patients and initiate a plan of care with assigned buddy that includes the shift's activities, feedback of care given, clinical and nursing care planning and intervention by the buddy, and establishment of priorities for care

5. Cosign physicians' orders and communicate those orders to assigned buddies and have other staff members initial orders after reading and understanding them

6. Maintain control of patient assignments when buddy is off the unit for any reason

If a nursing unit employs the buddy system, primary nurses may not have equal numbers of patients assigned. Again, assignments are based on the acuteness of illness and patient needs rather than on a number quotient. Fig. 5-4 is an example of an assignment sheet, which can be used to demonstrate the working relationship between buddies, primary and associate nurse compatibility, and how buddies cover for each other during the day such as at lunch time.

Buddies organize their daily plans to highlight comprehensive patient care and continuity of that care. Buddies begin their day by taking full patient reports on each other's patients. They formulate the nursing intervention to take place by either buddy throughout the day, including rounds with physicians, medications, and other patient care measures, and project a specific plan of care for the day during morning patient rounds, which the two buddies make together. Patients are introduced to each buddy, included in the planning of the day's activities, and familiarized with the day's procedures, tests, and treatments.

For example, on the day shift the morning begins with the nurses giving total patient care to their individual patients. The R.N. buddy cosigns physicians' orders for both sets of patients and communicates the orders to the auxiliary nurse, who initials the orders after reading and understanding them.

A specific feedback meeting time is established by the two buddies, and this meeting takes place before lunch break. At this time, buddies review their plans for patient care, which were formulated during early morning patient rounds, and concentrate their discussion on problem areas, general patient status, and evaluation of care given; an outline is then prepared for the afternoon plan of care. The head nurse can plan to attend these meetings as often as possible and, if not present for the discussions, should always receive the feedback either in verbal or written form.

The two buddies meet again in the afternoon to review and evaluate the care given to their patients during the day. If taped reports are utilized, buddies can report on their own patients after reviewing their reports with their buddies so that the most important, pertinent aspects of patient care are emphasized for the next shift.

Primary nurses select patients based on the ability of the nurse and the needs of the patient. It is important that units incorporating L.V.N.s into the primary nurse role devise a selection criteria that will clearly indicate to all levels of staff those patients the L.V.N. may consider selecting. For example, an R.N. might

* = Primary Nurse, x = Associate Nurse

UNIT: 3 SO.   DATE: 3/1   SHIFT: 7:30-3:30   CHARGE NURSE:

R.N. Nurse A	L.V.N. Nurse B	R.N. Nurse C	N.A. Nurse D	R.N. Nurse E	N.A. Nurse F	R.N. Nurse G	ADDITIONAL ASSIGNMENTS
*305A	*307A	*308A	*309A	*310A	*312A	*301	Emergency Equipment: A
* B	*	* B	* B	* B	* B	*302	Dressing Cart: B
x306A	x C	x C	x C	x311A	x313A	*303	I.V. Tray: C
x B	x D	x D	x315	x B	x B	x304	Medications Room: G
					x314		Conference Room: D
							Treatment Room: E
							Linen: F
LUNCH:							
12:00	11:30	11:30	11:00	12:30	12:00	12:30	

IN-SERVICE

1:00-1:30, Dr. Smith, "Death and Dying"

1:30-2:00, Patient-centered Conference, Nurse G

Fig. 5-4. Daily patient assignment using the buddy system.

select patients admitted for major surgeries, acute illnesses, multiple medications, intravenous feedings, major teaching areas, and major emotional and psychological problems. The L.V.N. might select patients admitted for minor surgeries, diagnostic tests, follow-through teaching in areas in which the nurse is knowledgeable, and chronic illnesses.

Reservations about giving the responsibility of primary nursing care to L.V.N.s are certainly reasonable, and it may not always be possible to continue an L.V.N. in a primary nursing role.

The primary nurse-patient relationship might have to be interrupted if the patient's status changes, no matter how many controls there are (such as selection criteria) or how much primary nursing promises continuous care to one patient by one nurse. An L.V.N. might select a patient admitted for minor surgery. If the patient's course continues as planned, there will be no interruption of care. However, if the patient's status changes for the worse, because of preoperative or postoperative complications, it would be in the patient's best interests clinically to change primary nurses. This aspect of primary nursing is no different from other delivery care systems that incorporate all levels of staff; this situation simply has to be expected by the staff when considering primary nursing.

SPECIAL TOOLS THAT PROMOTE PATIENTS' INVOLVEMENT IN THEIR CARE

There is continual and pressing concern to promote patients' participation in planning and evaluating their nursing care. Undoubtedly more tools are constantly being developed to further this effort. Primary nursing, as a patient care delivery system, certainly promotes this concept. Self-medication programs and group patient teaching are presently being experimented with in some hospitals across the country and will be discussed later in this chapter. Another way of involving patients in the evaluation of their care is to permit them to document and evaluate their care through recordings that are maintained by the patient.

Self-medication programs. It is typical that patients in the controlled environment of the hospital often ask few questions about their medications. When questions are posed, they tend to be more related to the name of the medication than to its use, toxicity, side effects, and results of improper use. Because of lack of education by nurses and/or physicians, patients are often discharged from the hospital with several prescriptions and little knowledge of what to expect from the medications. Readmissions resulting from improperly taken medications at home are not infrequent.

Patients on hospital self-medication programs can be trained and educated to properly take their medications after they have been discharged from the hospital. Furthermore, patients can achieve the maximum independence and reliability in self-administration of medications to ensure a minimum of dosage errors and maximum potentiality of continued and accurate medication administration. Primary nurses are the ideal persons to implement such programs.

Not all patients will qualify for a self-medication program; therefore patient selection criteria should be established by nursing units that are considering the program. A history of drug abuse, suicidal tendencies, a lack of motivation and desire to participate, and the lack of a minimal level of physical and mental ability (that is, the patient neither understands nor follows directions) are some disqualifying factors.

It is entirely possible that some patients may be disqualified to continue on the program. Changes in physical and mental conditions can be contributing factors. Inability to take medication properly and follow directions for its use are also reasons for terminating the patient in the program. It is therefore necessary to ensure that continual evaluation of patients and their ability to understand and assimilate the program takes place.

Coordination of the self-medication program for a primary patient is facilitated through the communication triangle, which includes physician, head nurse, and primary nurse. The primary nurse interviews and assesses the patient and discusses the assessment with the physician and head nurse. If the patient is selected for the program, the primary nurse explains the objectives, methods, importance of charting, and directions for administering medications to the patient. Narcotics, hypnotics, and barbiturates are generally excluded from self-medication programs because of federal control laws. It is generally considered the safest policy to contain the patient's medications in a locked repository at the bedside, out of sight and reach of other patients and visitors.

The primary nurse must closely supervise and monitor the patient's self-administered medications for the first several days during the program. As the patient demonstrates the ability to comprehend and take the responsibility for administering medications, an independent status for self-administration can begin; that is, the patient can be allowed to begin independent administration, charting and retaining medications at the bedside.

The patient assumes the responsibility for charting medications. The name of the drug, dosage, time, route of administration, and use is recorded on the sheet by the primary nurse. As medications, dosage, and times change or are discontinued, the changes are reflected on the sheet by the primary nurse. Fig. 5-5 is an example of a patient self-medication record that can be kept at the patient's bedside. The patient documents the time each medication is taken and initials the time. The record is incorporated into the patient's chart each week, and a new sheet is given to the patient. Prior to discharge, patients can be given records to take home with them to foster continuing accuracy of self-administration after discharge from the hospital.

Medications are counted on a daily basis to ensure that the correct amount is taken. During the patient's first days on the program, the primary nurse and patient count together. For example, if a patient receives ten pills of digoxin, 125 mg. each, from the pharmacy and is to take one a day, there will be one less pill each day. At the bottom of the patient's self-medication record is an area designated for the medication count. The patient continues the count for the remainder of the hospitalization and is encouraged to continue the count after discharge from the hospital. Patients are also instructed to alert the nurse and physician of symptoms, side effects, and any adverse reactions from the medication. A patient profile record can be utilized by patients to record their observations of the effects of medication, comments on the program, and comments on their individual progress as a result of the program. The patient profile record in Fig. 5-6 not only

Medication, Dosage, Time Route of Administration, and Use	3/1	3/2	3/3	3/4	3/5	3/6
Digoxin .25 mgm. daily Oral, 9:00 A.M., for heart	9 A.m. AC Pulse · 72	9 A M. AC Pulse-80	9 A.m. AC Pulse· 76			
Lasix 20 mgm. daily Oral, 9:00 A.M., for edema	9 A.M AC	9 A.M AC	9 A.M. AC			
ASA gr X every 4 hrs. as necessary, Oral, for headache		7A.M. AC				
MEDICATION COUNT:						
Digoxin .23 mgm (10)	9	8	7			
Lasix 20 mgm (10)	9	8	7			
ASA gr V (10)		8				

Fig. 5-5. Patient self-medication record.

MEDICATION	COMMENTS (effect, side effects, adverse reactions)

DATE	PATIENT Evaluation of Program and Individual Progress

Fig. 5-6. Patient profile record.

provides an excellent evaluation tool for the patient but also aids the nurse and physician in evaluating and assessing the patient's continuing comprehension of the program.

Prior to discharge the primary nurse again reviews all discharge medications, their use, and time of administration with the patient and family. The patient is again alerted to notify the physician concerning side effects or any problems with the medications.

Group patient teaching. Most patients are instructed at some time during their hospitalization by nurses concerning their illness, surgery, medications, treatment, or other aspects of their care. Because individual instruction can be time consuming, alternatives must be available for both nurses and patients to facilitate a greater, more comprehensive teaching-learning environment. At the same time, group patient interaction can foster a highly therapeutic supportive milieu for patients in which anxieties and fears can be expressed and alleviated. Furthermore, group teaching can help decrease patient's feelings of isolation often experienced in the unfamiliar hospital setting.

Group instruction can be planned for primary patients with the same illnesses, surgeries, treatments, diets, and so on. There is ample evidence that group instruction has been successful with child care classes, community organizations, such as the colostomy clubs, and postoperative teaching. Group instruction on a nursing unit can also include family members to enhance the family's support and understanding during a member's illness.

Because units are becoming more specialized (that is, units with patients having similar illnesses), each unit is limited in the amount of group instruction it will be able to provide. On a surgical unit, for example, the emphasis will be preoperative and postoperative teaching, which can be either global or specific in approach.

The content of material to be taught during group instruction is coordinated with the nursing staff and the physicians on a particular unit. Because it is often at the physician's discretion whether the patient attends group sessions, the physician must understand the benefits of the teaching and exactly what the primary nurse will tell the patient.

An ideal way for primary nurses to organize group teaching is to include all their primary patients in the group. Usually there are commonalities among patients that can be surfaced and dealt with by the nurse. Primary nurses may have their patients located in the same physical locale of the unit such as the same room, in which case the patients may have already established a group process. Since the primary nurse has had close relationships with all the group members, pinpointing patient fears, apprehensions, and areas of ignorance is often easier. If these patients also have associate nurses, the primary nurse may wish to include the associate nurse as a co-teacher in the group.

Patient recordings. Patients can be given both the opportunity to participate in planning their care and the right to evaluate the care they receive. It is valuable to have patients' open-ended responses to what happens to them throughout their hospitalization. A patient's daily recordings can remind the nurse that the patient's opinions count a great deal, as well as give the nurse additional data for assessment of the patient's condition, and can alleviate the patient's feelings of helplessness in controlling what happens to him.

The patient must be told that his nurse will use his recordings in planning his care, and therefore he should record things that concern, puzzle, or irritate him. Usually patients are surprised that the nurse cares that much and are excited initially by the idea of a personal "diary." The novelty can wear off, however; therefore patients must be encouraged to continue their recordings, even though they might think "nothing" is happening to them.

Patient's Name _____

Room Number _____

Primary Nurse _____

Associate Nurse(s) _____

_____

Time/Date	What Happened	What I Thought and How I Felt
2:00 3/1	I came to the hospital and met my "primary nurse." She talked to me a long time about my care.	I was impressed that I will have my own nurse who will stay with me 'till I go home. I will have an "associate nurse" too—I wonder what she will be like.
5:00 3/1	My primary nurse spent a lot of time talking with me about my surgery.	I think I'm afraid of "going under the knife." My nurse will be there though. She assured me it was a "routine operation."
7:00 3/1	Tonight they got me ready for surgery—shaved me and stuff.	My nurse said they shave such a large area because they try to prevent infection—I'm sure glad she said that because I was afraid they were going to take out more than I thought.
9:00 3/1	My "associate nurse" gave me a strong sleeping pill and said I can't drink any water after midnight. She stayed and talked with me.	I feel really sleepy—I think I know what to expect. I'm glad my nurses take the time to describe everything to me.

Fig. 5-7. Patient recording form.

Fig. 5-7 is a sample patient recording form with comments that might be made by a preoperative male patient who does not want to undergo surgery. Such a form gives the patient an opportunity to vent his feelings but can be useful for other reasons as well. The patient can record minute-to-minute feelings and thoughts that help both the primary and associate nurse know what he is experiencing. Both nurses have a patient account of the previous shift. When the patient describes events and his thoughts and feelings, he often provides data that reveal how effective the teaching has been and that alert the nurse to other patient needs or desires.

SUGGESTED READINGS

Doctor's business: Indiana nurses reject four-day week, Medical World News, Dec. 3, 1971.

Kent, L. A.: The 4-40 workweek on trial, American Journal of Nursing 72:683-686, 1972.

Kramer, M.: Standard 4—nursing care plans—power to the patient, Journal of Nursing Administration, pp. 29-34, Sept.-Oct., 1972.

Little, D. E., and Carnevali, D. L.: Communicating by means of nursing care plans. In Nursing care planning, Philadelphia, 1969, J. B. Lippincott, Co., pp. 187-204.

Mezzanotte, E. J.: Group instruction in preparation for surgery, American Journal of Nursing **70:**89-91, 1970.

Morse, J.: Second thoughts on the 4-day work week, Oakland Tribune, Dec. 24, 1972.

Pohl, M. L.: Teaching function of the nursing practitioner, Dubuque, 1968, William C. Brown Co.

Price, E. M.: Staffing for patient care, New York, 1970, Springer Publishing Co.

chapter 6

PROCESSES OF CHANGE NECESSARY TO IMPLEMENT PRIMARY NURSING

The ability to introduce change with a minimum of resistance is a key management skill. It requires the change agent to understand the impact of decisions made and the effect these changes will have on the personnel involved. But most important, it requires employees to be informed about why the change is being made and to be involved in the actual decision-making process. According to Gilbert,[1] employees involved in the change are more likely to take an active interest in the work situation and more likely to take responsibility for the outcomes of the change process. By definition, "planned change" implies collaboration and cooperative endeavor. This process of changing is a process of choice and is distinctly different from change that occurs by indoctrination, accident, coercion, or growth (natural).[2]

Several bridges must be crossed before primary nursing can be fully implemented. This chapter will attempt to identify key steps in easing the entire implementation process. These are (1) preparing for change by acknowledging the need for change and by defining the parameters for change, (2) scheduling and implementing the change at the unit level, and (3) maintaining and evaluating the change according to specified criteria.

PREPARING FOR CHANGE

Perhaps the most difficult and yet the most important phase of planned change is the preparation for the change itself. In preparing for change the first glimpse of vast uncharted territory awakens fear and anxiety in the change agents. The vagueness of what is to be done and who is to do it can be overwhelming, enough so to discourage those who are currently seeking improvements to give up any ideas of changing. The preparation phase is crucial, since it is here that many plans are delayed from even "getting off the drawing board." The following discussion describes two important subordinate tasks of this stage that must be mastered before proceeding to actual implementation. They are (1) acknowledging the need for change and establishing administrative commitment and (2) defining the parameters for change by redefinition of key roles.

Acknowledging the need for change and establishing administrative commitment

Key organizational people must support and participate in the change.[2] Although the decision to implement primary nursing may be provoked by staff, it ultimately rests with the administration's perception of the need for a change. The decision to implement primary nursing is based on the administration's acknowledgement that there are more ways, and perhaps better ways, to deliver nursing care than those currently employed. Purveyors of health services are always looking for better ways to deliver nursing care that are more cost-effective, more goal-effective, and more patient-centered. Planned change in the area of dispensing nursing care is change with a purpose. Primary nursing is a solution to the need for change because standard procedures and organization cannot cope. Understanding that primary nursing is such a system is essential. Primary nursing has a goal and projects methods to attain that goal. As a system it is goal oriented and has definite components that fit together so that the system can be realized and that a better nursing modality can be obtained.

The administrator must understand that primary nursing is also capable of fostering personal and professional growth for the nurse, and this is an important ingredient to justify the change. The administrator's communication of his commitment to individualized patient care and his eagerness to explore the effects of new nursing care modalities is tantamount to ensuring the implementation, maintenance, and ultimate success of primary nursing. His commitment must be communicated not only to the nurses, who will experiment with the change, but also to physicians and department heads who may be directly or indirectly affected by the change. Questions, problems, and praise from the patient, physician, and nursing service go first to the administrator's office. The administrator by articulating his commitment will be able to explain the benefits he expects as a result of the change. He may vary his explanations but will almost always mention his expectations for a highly satisfied nursing staff and highly satisfied patients receiving individualized and personalized care.

Physicians, particularly those participating in administrative capacities, have tremendous influence in setting standards for patient care. To stimulate and support the steps necessary for implementation of the changes, physicians must be directly involved in the planning and implementation of the changes. They must know how primary nursing will affect patients, as well as its implications in terms of their own roles. They must be told that the total nursing care of the patient will be the responsibility of one nurse, who will know a great deal about the patient, and that it will be the primary nurse and not the head nurse who will answer many of the physicians' questions.

Physicians are an important group to nurses, and they need to be included in planning, in the feedback circuit and in the in-service education of primary nurses. This in turn will produce a colleagueship of health care delivery. As the system matures and the payoff becomes obvious, physicians also get the glow of pride and reinforcement that comes from sharing this colleagueship. Good planning relationships with physicians then feed back into the system and cause nurses and physicians to work cooperatively for personalized patient care.

Defining the parameters for change by redefinition of key roles

Inherent in change and in the implementation of primary nursing is the redefinition of the roles of personnel affected by the change. Redefinition of roles makes the anticipated change appear concrete and tangible and can allay some of the anxieties of personnel about what the change will mean to them as individuals. Because acceptance is often the result of understanding, nursing personnel need to understand both the expectations of their roles and their participation in describing the changes. How key staff become involved in change and how their roles may change because of primary nursing implementation are described in the following discussion of the roles of the director of nursing, supervisor, and head nurse. The roles of the primary nurse and other unit-level personnel were discussed in Chapters 4 and 5 and will be discussed later in this chapter.

Director of nursing. Before selecting a nursing care modality that fits their situations and needs, directors of nursing must investigate and become informed about a variety of nursing care modalities. When a mode such as primary nursing is chosen, each director will then need to pursue a self-educational program of reading, investigation, and discussion with other directors to assess the requirements of primary nursing. After becoming better informed, the director is able to take the steps necessary to make primary nursing work effectively.

The director of nursing is the central figure in determining the direction and the quality of patient care and the character of the director–staff nurse relationship. There are two inherent aspects of the role of the director: leadership in influencing quality patient care and administrative functioning. A director with only an administrative role can critically impede improvement of nursing care and ultimately affect nursing leadership. The director who is confined solely to administrative responsibilities tends to neglect the role of planning and evaluating nursing services. According to Sheehan,[3] assigning the director a nonnursing director who would become responsible for administrative and nonnursing functions enables the director to function in a purely nursing leadership capacity.

The director's role in primary nursing parallels the administrator's commitment for individualized patient care and reinforces this attitude with the rest of the hospital. The director's commitment to primary nursing directly affects the roles and attitudes of nurses involved in giving patient care.

The director understands the organization and the expectations for primary nursing, which includes how patients should be treated and how staff should perform. Regularly scheduled meetings with both the supervisor and head nurse of the primary nursing unit can establish a feedback system for discussion of progress and problems of planning, implementing, and maintaining the change. Meetings that include all hospital supervisors and head nurses and that are held on a regular basis further encourage a stimulating growth-oriented hospital environment in which experiences are shared and change is "everybody's business."

The director of nursing reinforces primary nursing with physicians and other hospital personnel. By maintaining a feedback system with these groups, the director positively reinforces their participation in the change and gains important insight into how other departments are affected by primary nursing implementation.

Being patient-centered and staff development–oriented requires more than stating it. Staff nurses are no longer satisfied with "lip service" from nursing service and want tangible evidence that their nursing leaders support them. As the role model for nursing leadership and the spokesman for the top corporate structure, the director's involvement at the unit level is essential. The director can convey a commitment to nursing units and thereby affect quality nursing care standards in several ways. The interaction of the director with the unit should include making unit rounds, conducting patient and staff interviews, and becoming directly involved in unit problems. Probably one of the more important purposes of the director's interaction with staff on the unit is to give reinforcement for small successes.

Sometimes when struggling with change, it is easier to see the problems inherent in change, rather than the successes, because the people involved are so anxious about the change. When people on the top of the corporate structure can recognize even small successes and feed that recognition and praise back into the system, it is highly stimulating for the staff and instrumental in continuing the change process. Staff members are not only encouraged but also motivated to continue efforts.

Directors need to communicate not only support but also encouragement to staff members to experiment. They must make the structure flexible enough to allow for experimentation. For example, one director in a midwest hospital told her supervisor to take as long as necessary to develop her role and gave her the time to do so. The important aspect here is to match verbal support with action, that is, time and resources to accomplish the experiment. The director provides more than "lip service" by understanding that commitment for implementation of change must be matched with opportunities to take the steps to change and that each step must be reinforced as a small but significant success.

Supervisor. The supervisor's role may well be the most nebulous role in the primary nursing system. Some hospitals have deleted the role altogether, whereas others are changing the title and at the same time changing the functions of the role. There seems to be some general agreement, however, that supervisors can operate in ways that enhance primary nursing. Clearly evident is the role of supervisor as a clinical expert and resource for primary nurses, who need a nursing care consultant for specific problems. Second, the supervisor can act as a communication channel between the director of nursing and the head nurse, especially in those hospitals in which direct communication between the director and head nurse is missing. More appropriate to primary nursing, however, is the supervisor who can supplement rather than replace the communication between the director and head nurse. Finally, the supervisor can collaborate with the head nurse to enhance staff development while enacting her role of resource person.

The supervisor's role is complementary to the head nurse's role. Supervisors need to be knowledgeable concerning staff members' capabilities and limitations to provide constructive guidelines and positive reinforcement for staff members. At the same time the supervisor is involved in planning, implementing, and evaluating primary nursing and must be aware of the objectives of this kind of unit.

Understanding the head nurse's expectations for the unit, the unit nursing care standards, staff development goals, and performance criteria is essential for the supervisor. Periodic attendance at patient reports and selected patient rounds by the supervisor provides an overview of patient problems, as well as an opportunity to give recognition to staff for their performance. The supervisor by acting as a resource person and clinical role model for staff can be involved in problem solving on a one-to-one basis with staff members and thus foster a broader perspective for staff members engaged in nursing assessments.

The supervisor's continued commitment to the unit's objectives can be reflected by her enthusiastic participation in staff meetings, in-service meetings, and other conferences in which modalities of patient care delivery are discussed. The supervisor and head nurse need to meet regularly and discuss their ideas about unit coordination, staff performance, and quality patient care standards. By providing guidelines and tools for continued unit growth and development, the supervisor helps the unit achieve independence in the same way that head nurses develop independent primary nurses.

The supervisor can be the only communication link between the director of nursing and the head nurse or can supplement this communication pattern. Especially in larger hospitals, it can be difficult for the director to meet regularly with every head nurse, even though very often the door is open to head nurses. Because communication can be changed as it travels through channels, there is frequently less misrepresentation if the communication is direct. Direct communication with the director sometimes provides a more efficient way to resolve and solve problems and intensifies the collaborative effort between the director of nursing and the head nurse. However, depending on the specific hospital and the availability of the director, direct communication is sometimes impractical.

In addition, the director of nursing, the supervisor, and the head nurse have different positions and different functions, and make different observations of the patient care given and received. These three people collaborating and communicating their differences together can highlight and bring into perspective patient care needs and objectives—outcomes that are sometimes more fruitful than that of communication between only head nurse and director or between only the head nurse and the supervisor.

An important issue arising from the supervisor's role is the problem of territory. Although some hospitals continue to make supervisors responsible for all hospitalized patients, other hospitals are assigning supervisors to specific areas of the hospital. For example, an acute care supervisor may be responsible for the intensive care unit, the coronary care unit, and the respiratory care unit. Another supervisor is perhaps responsible for all medical-surgical units. Some hospitals have defined and implemented two separate supervisory roles to oversee the entire hospital: administrative supervisors and clinical supervisors. With respect to primary nursing care, we can envision supervisors specifically assigned to those units that are primary nursing units. No matter how the services of the hospital are arranged, one point is worth noting: if hospitals continue to utilize supervisors, they need to be readily accessible to nursing units as nursing care consultants for specific patient problems. Their accessibility is increased and their knowledge is better communicated if the number of units or specialties that they are assigned are kept to a minimum. Administrative responsibilities heretofore taken on by a clinically oriented supervisor should not be overseen by this clinical specialist.

Head nurse. The head nurse role can be delineated to include the following functions—quality control agent, validator, nursing care coordinator and resource, facilitator of staff development and growth, and communication channel both upward and downward. Manthey[4] describes the head nurse role as the most important determinant in ensuring the success of primary nursing. She perceives the head nurse as providing strong leadership, motivation, staff development, and clinical assessment.

Crucial to the head nurse's role, as well as to the supervisor's or director's role, is the old proverb, "Know thyself." Head nurses threatened by change, by innovative staff members, or, for that matter, by hospital hierarchy will be insecure, making and affecting decisions that are not germane to either patient care or staff development. Head nurses who have clear objectives and who realize that growth is a shared experience for all personnel will make and affect decisions that will be pertinent. Their role will prove to be important in ensuring the success of both change and growth for the staff.

As a quality control agent the head nurse is directly accountable for both patient care and staff development on a twenty-four–hour basis. In addition to hearing full patient shift report, the head nurse makes complete daily patient rounds. The head nurse fosters a unit environment in which both staff and patient problems can be expressed and solved as they occur and while they are relevant.

The head nurse comprehensively assesses each nurse and knows the specific capabilities and limitations of all staff members. At the same time the head nurse assists each staff member to select primary patients concurrent with the staff nurse's abilities. Provisions for further development of clinical skills is accomplished through unit in-service programs.

The head nurse treats staff members as accountable for patient care and builds this accountability in several ways. Scheduling of primary nurses, expecting primary nurses to select and follow through on primary patients, and expecting a single professional standard for performance are some ways the head nurse reinforces staff accountability.

The head nurse can ensure that quality patient care standards are achieved by implementing unit nursing audits and performance evaluations as well as comparing standards and performance with measurements from formal research. At the same time appropriate changes can be made, thus enhancing quality patient care and staff performance.

The head nurse as a validator is the person with whom staff nurses can check out and validate their plans. In primary nursing the primary nurse is expected to assess the patient comprehensively and then to initiate and continue a twenty-four–hour plan of care based on this assessment. Primary nurses prior to initiating the care plan check their assessments with the head nurse. The head nurse as the chief resource person for the staff can assist the nurse by examining the data gathered and by collaborating with the primary nurse to organize a relevant and workable care plan. The primary nurse continues to reevaluate the patient's plan of care throughout his hospitalization, reflecting changes and updating the nursing care plan. In addition, the primary nurse continues to check out and validate these observations with the head nurse.

Primary nurses also validate their plans for self-development with the head nurse. Again, the primary nurse and head nurse examine and discuss the staff member's experience, education, and aspirations and then construct a relevant and workable plan of self-enhancement for the nurse.

As nursing care coordinators, head nurses are the unit role models for viewing patients and demonstrate the expertise of their knowledge and experience through their holistic approach to patient-centered care. Because primary nurses often emulate the head nurse, it is implicit in the head nurse role to recognize and trust the patient as the central figure in planning care. The head nurse coordinates all other services and personnel with the patient remaining as the focus.

As the nursing care coordinator, the head nurse synchronizes the three nursing shifts so that staff on the different shifts harmonize their objectives for patient care and their subsequent nursing actions. The head nurse also coordinates the activities and objectives for each shift in terms of its uniqueness from the other shifts.

The head nurse coordinates hospital objectives and policies with unit objectives and policies. Improved quality patient care standards, patient safety, and improved nursing performance standards are outgrowths of this effort.

Perhaps the chief responsibility of the head nurse is to facilitate staff growth and development. Head nurses can no longer focus solely on the patient to affect quality patient care. Only when the nurse caring for the patient is receiving quality, individualized direction will the patient begin to obtain the quality, individualized, patient-centered care that nursing needs to promise.

On a primary nursing unit the head nurse recognizes the primary nurse as accountable for patient care planning and delivery. The head nurse also understands that primary nurses need to be highly knowledgeable practitioners who can be self-motivated, innovative, and independent in providing patient-centered care. But to accept accountability and to practice independently, primary nurses must have readily accessible tools that will enhance their growth and development. The head nurse as the facilitator for development provides and coordinates educational and experiential opportunities for individuals as well as for the group.

Providing individual staff development means that the head nurse initiates and continues a dialogue with each staff member. Inherent in the dialogue is mutual understanding of growth opportunities and areas that need improvement. The head nurse and staff nurse collaborate on an individual plan for development that is positive and relevant for the nurse. It is important that the head nurse give positive reinforcement for the nurse's abilities during the dialogue.

The head nurse can offer the primary nurse multiple resources for problem solving and individual development. Appropriate hospital and community in-service programs can be recommended to the nurse. The head nurse or supervisor can be utilized for patient observations and clinical problem solving. Conferences between the primary nurse and the unit in-service coordinator can produce relevant suggestions that can help the staff nurse resolve any limitations. The head nurse can also delegate responsibilities that are concurrent with the nurse's individual objectives, such as leading in-service projects, being accountable for unit staff scheduling, assuming a charge position, or developing more relevant tools for staff members within primary nursing.

Inherent in the dialogue is the fact the primary nurses are encouraged to identify their own problems and to become part of the decision-making process that will affect both their attitudes and growth. By doing this, the head nurse fosters a constructive attitude for change with the primary nurse. Documentation of the counseling can provide a basis for future evaluation as well as reinforcement for progress.

Management, which in this case is the head nurse, can accomplish change by effectively communicating the need for change and by stimulating group participation in planning the changes. Implicit in group development is staff recognition within the group. The keynote in promoting a colleague relationship is the fact that within the group there are individuals who have personal and professional objectives for themselves. The head nurse fosters a cohesive peer group that can identify and solve staff problems within the group. By problem solving and participative management, objectives can be described for the group, with a focus emerging that is constructive and relevant, rather than one divided by dissident factions interposed by personality factors.

Head nurses are also the central unit channels for communication, both upward and downward. They communicate hospital plans, objectives, and policies to their staff, as well as communicate staff objectives and plans to nursing administration. They do not simply disseminate information but question, appraise, collaborate, and support the communciation after a final decision is made.

As an integral part of the communication triangle, the head nurse participates as a colleague with primary nurses and physicians in discussing, planning, and evaluating patient care. To highlight the physician–primary nurse colleagueship, the head nurse can defer physician inquiries to the primary nurse and receive feedback from them after their discussions.

In summary, as the quality control agent, validator, nursing care coordinator, and facilitator for growth and development, the head nurse is the role model for primary nurses and communicates quality patient care standards, nursing performance standards, and standards for growth and development to them. The head nurse also communicates and fosters an environment in which people are important. The outgrowth of this kind of a milieu is nurses who are responsive to change, encouraged by constructive criticism, and motivated by their individual as well as group development.

On a primary nursing unit the head nurse will see a different reward system emerge. Reward systems presently are designed with bureaucratic ideals in mind. Primary nursing, however, shifts to a humanistic reward system in which primary nurses are rewarded by seeing their patients get better care and better assessments. The nurse's plans and actions pay off in happier and healthier humans. The head nurse is seen as a collaborator and no longer as a policeman and record keeper. Human relationships and colleagueships evolve with patients and with each other as they collaborate and validate planning. This shift from bureaucracy to humanism is a necessary shift and the reinforcing factor that will make the primary nursing system thrive in the hospital setting.

SCHEDULING AND IMPLEMENTING THE CHANGE

Having acknowledged the need for change and specified the roles of key organizational participants, the actual scheduling and implementation of change becomes an important activity for staff. Although it may be a relatively straightforward and easy task, there are important points to keep in mind.

It is essential for the head nurse, supervisor, and director to have a well-defined plan for implementation, involving all personnel affected by change. If the rate of implementation occurs in a time sequence that is gauged to the ability of the staff to assimilate change, a smoother operation will result. The establishment of target dates and objectives around timing realities enables staff to pace their achievements realistically.[5]

Short-term as well as long-term objectives should be clearly defined and understood. As objectives are achieved, positive reinforcement can be given to promote further motivation to bring about the intended change. Concomitant to this is the task of redefining the roles of staff involved in the change, establishing performance criteria, and having tools available to measure and maintain the change.

Planning for implementation and the implementation process for primary nursing involve several steps as indicated in the following suggested method.

    A. Ground work

        1. Provide staff, physicians, and appropriate department heads with primary nursing reading lists. Schedule group discussions to review the material to foster a comprehensive working knowledge of primary nursing.

    2. Provide unit in-service meetings on the dynamics of problem solving, communication lines, primary nursing interviews, histories and physicals, primary nursing care plans, discharge planning, and home visits.

    3. Discuss in detail role changes and performance criteria.

    4. Provide staff members with the opportunity to role play primary and associate nurses' roles and interview techniques.

    5. Discuss in detail evaluation tools to be used.

B. Implementation at the unit level

    1. Tape shift reports and include all staff in listening to reports. Allow staff members to report on their own patients.

    2. Assign patients on a total patient care basis. Each nurse assumes full responsibility for patient care within that assignment, which includes administering medication and treatment, cosigning physicians' orders, bathing, changing linens, and other tasks.

    3. Initiate the buddy system if this is appropriate to the unit and evaluate daily communication between nurses and decisions based on assessments.

    4. Initiate Kardex rounds and patient-centered conferences with all levels of staff participating.

    5. Initiate selection of primary patients one shift at a time, although nurses may opt to select when they think they are ready. Initiate associate nurse status when appropriate.

    6. As progress of the unit's adaptability to the change becomes evident, set a goal for when all patients will be selected.

    7. Utilize evaluation tools to measure accurately and to maintain the change.

    8. Continue in-service meetings, with emphasis on problem areas for staff.

To reiterate, primary nursing is gradually implemented with full understanding of staff, physicians, supportive personnel, and patients. Implementation occurs at intervals at which time progress is evidenced and reinforced. The time sequence needed for each step will be dependent on the unit and the institution. Progressive hospitals with action-oriented nursing leaders, who are continually evaluating and upgrading quality patient care standards, are familiar with change. They can implement changes swiftly and with little resistance. On the other hand, hospitals making infrequent changes will encounter more resistance, and the implementation process may need to be more gradual.

MAINTAINING AND EVALUATING THE CHANGE

Evaluation is frequently thought of as a terminating event. With primary nursing and the institution of planned change, evaluation occurs at every stage of development as follows: (1) at the onset when a need for change is recognized, (2) at the time when implementation occurs so that the plan for change is realistic, and (3) at a more advanced stage when staff members hope to maintain and get reinforcement for the successes they have had. The following discussion of maintenance and evaluation tools includes a description of performance criteria that may used to evaluate staff and explanations of how staff evaluations, care plans, nursing audits, formal research, and staff meetings and workshops can be utilized to maintain and evaluate primary nursing.

Establishing performance criteria

When performance criteria are established, the nurse must understand and be a part of the decision-making process that defines the expectations for performance. The traditional criterion of grooming and punctuality as indicators of efficiency are not germane to primary nursing. Efficiency really means to achieve objectives in the most effective manner with the least amount of investment of time, energy, and money. Unit objectives for primary nursing are discussed in Chapter 4 and provide the basis for the performance criteria to be described here. The key objective for performance in primary nursing is to provide individualized patient care. The primary nurse is accountable for the twenty-four–hour plan of care for specific patients. Continuance of this care occurs with associate nurses. The head nurse enhances each nurse's capabilities and awareness to deal with patients through staff development.

Delineation of the key objective for primary nursing provides staff members specific guidelines for performance. All criteria that follow are in behavioral terms, that is, they state what the staff nurse should do. Nonbehavioral criteria are avoided because they do not lead to observation and measurement.

The primary nurse is directly accountable for planning, communicating, and evaluating care for primary patients on a twenty-four–hour basis and for the duration of the patient's hospitalization. More specifically, the nurse's responsibilities are as follows:

1. To select and remain accountable for two or more primary patients at all times
2. To identify the primary nurse's role to patients, physicians, family, and staff
3. To select, plan, and evaluate patient care with associate nurses
4. To initiate and complete the primary nursing interview, history, and physical on admission of the patient
5. To initiate and design a twenty-four–hour primary nursing care plan, continuing to reflect any changes on the care plan based on communication with the physician and associate nurses
6. To reflect pertinent observations on the Kardex so that other staff are alerted to highlights of the patient's comprehensive needs
7. To give total comprehensive patient care
8. To maintain and coordinate the communication triangle between physician, head nurse, and primary nurse
9. To initiate patient-centered conferences to coordinate the patient's care with the entire staff
10. To initiate discharge planning at the time of admission and to continue plans for discharge during the patient's hospitalization

11. To utilize and coordinate community agencies and other resources
12. To provide continuity of care by evaluating patients for home visits and by making home visits when appropriate

The associate nurse is accountable for providing continuity of care to the primary nurse's patients. Associate nurses are scheduled for shifts different from the primary nurse and follow up the patient throughout hospitalization. Associate nurses can also be scheduled to work the same shift as the primary nurse in the primary nurse's absence. It is important to understand that primary nurses can be both primary and associate nurses. For example, a primary nurse may be primary for two patients and associate for several patients as discussed in Chapter 4. More specifically, the associate nurse's responsibilities are as follows:

1. To accept and/or select to provide continuity of care planned by the primary nurse
2. To identify the associate nurse's role to patients, physicians, family, and staff
3. To provide continuity of care as planned by the primary nurse and maintain communication with the primary nurse concerning care
4. To reflect changes on the primary nursing care plan based on observations, assessments, and communication with the patient and physician in the primary nurse's absence
5. To reflect pertinent observations on the Kardex
6. To give total comprehensive patient care
7. To participate in the communication triangle with the physician and head nurse in the primary nurse's absence
8. To participate or to initiate patient-centered conferences to enhance continuity of care for the entire staff
9. To continue discharge planning as coordinated by the primary nurse

Staff development is implicit on a primary nursing unit. Hospital nursing units, although becoming more specialized, still have basic attitudes in common toward development. Although highly specialized units (such as intensive care and coronary care units) would probably want to include specific criteria for their units, the following list of criteria not only identifies for staff the attitude necessary for development but specifically describes resources available for growth.

1. To define and accept unit objectives and performance criteria
2. To identify self-capabilities and limitations and to collaborate with the head nurse to produce an individual plan for development
3. To accept constructive criticism related to performance and attitude and to demonstrate acceptance by appropriate changes
4. To positively reinforce co-workers' capabilities
5. To give constructive criticism related to performance and attitude
6. To promote a cohesive work environment
7. To promote peer review
8. To participate in the decision-making process, both individually and on a group level

9. To identify areas for expanded growth
10. To identify growth opportunities in shift rotation
11. To attend staff meetings and workshops
12. To attend community workshops

The processes of problem solving are an integral part of the entire ciriteria. Problem solving leads to decision making, and without it effective decision making would not take place. Problem solving is utilized by nurses in all aspects of patient care as well as by nursing leaders. All staff members, especially primary and associate nurses, should be able to (1) consider a broad analysis of problems; (2) consider multiple resources and sources of information; (3) consider alternative interventions; (4) assign priorities to problems and interventions; (5) review the consequences of alternative interventions; (6) make decisions based on conclusions formulated from the previous process; (7) implement a plan for intervention; and (8) evaluate the results of the intervention as a basis for further growth and development.

Questionnaires administered to all staff members can serve as an effective and efficient tool for assessing the group's general expectations and for initiating a performance criteria that is relevant and acceptable to staff. Volunteers from the unit can serve on a professional performance committee to establish general guidelines. Staff meetings can be scheduled by the committee to promote full involvement of the staff in describing the specific expectations for the criteria. Head nurses and supervisors can establish criteria relevant to their roles in a similar manner.

Evaluation of the employee, then, is a measurement against the performance criteria. A single rather than a double standard emerges for patient care and staff performance. Nurses know specifically what is expected of them and that they will be measured against those expectations. They will not be evaluated on the basis of personality factors but on the basis of their performance in the areas described in the criteria.

In primary nursing performance criteria are essential. Roles change, and the need for clarification within those roles is important for the nurse. With primary nursing, responsibilities and accountability for nursing care changes. Without specific guidelines for performance, nurses can become highly frustrated and overwhelmed by new expectations placed on them.

Additional tools for maintenance and evaluation of change

In addition to performance criteria, several measurement tools are available in primary nursing to evaluate and maintain change. These tools include staff evaluations, primary nursing care plans, nursing audits, and formal research. By utilizing evaluation tools, the staff and nursing administration can accurately appraise staff performance, patient care standards, and the patient's perceptions of the care received. In addition, regularly scheduled staff meetings and staff workshops increase staff communication and allow staff members formalized periods to evaluate their performance.

Staff evaluations. Staff evaluations are effective when performance is appraised at regular intervals, and, during these evaluations, progress and problems are communicated. A six-month evaluation conference, which occurs between the head nurse and each staff member, is more pertinent for the primary nurse. This conference includes an overview of the staff member's performance, and the evaluation is supplemented with anecdotal notes written in the interim that document specific progress or problems.

Head nurses can maintain, in addition to the hospital personnel files, staff evaluation and progress files on the unit. The unit files can serve as a basis for comparison of progress for the head nurse and the primary nurse. They are readily available to either person for purposes of evaluation or for initiating a plan of development for the staff nurse based on performance. These files could be incorporated into the hospital files on a yearly basis.

Included in the unit files can be anecdotal notes concerning interim performance, unit in-service activities, continuance of formal education, questionnaires, areas of special recognition, and six-month evaluations. Maintaining the files is a cooperative effort between the head nurse, assistant head nurse, and the unit in-service coordinator. The files are available to all staff members as well as supervisory personnel. Maintaining unit files can foster an environment in which performing at one's highest capabilities is emphasized, rather than "getting by" with mediocre yet passable performance.

Anecdotal notes can be written by any employee concerning the performance of another employee. Anecdotes can also be written by employees concerning their own performance. In addition to promoting peer review, anecdotal notes document specific performance and provide immediate feedback to employees concerning their performance. Anecdotal notes can include demonstrated problem-solving ability, primary nurse–patient relationships, leadership ability, and interstaff relationships and give specific accounts of the nurse's performance. In addition to giving the written anecdotal note to the head nurse, the nurse writing the note should share it with the staff member observed. The feedback received by the nurse includes positive reinforcement for ability of counseling when there are problems. The employee then has the opportunity to improve problem areas before receiving the six-month performance evaluation. Finally, problems can be handled at a level of constructive dialogue.

Documentation by the in-service coordinator on those employees taking active parts in leading in-service projects can be kept in each nurse's file. Conferences attended as well as continuing formal education can also be recorded.

Special recognition can include letters from patients, teaching or speaking with the hospital or community, awards received relating to personal or professional growth, and published material. Questionnaires received from staff, especially those involving areas of improvement needed by the nurse, can be kept and reviewed by the head nurse and unit leaders to ensure that these improvement needs are being met. Yearly performance evaluations are required by most hospitals and serve as a recommendation for the employee for future jobs. They also serve as a guideline for the employee during employment in the current hospital. Six-month performance evaluations are recommended to provide the nurse with more pertinent data on performance and in doses more easily assimilated. Once criteria for performance are established, an evaluation tool to measure the nurse against these criteria is more easily developed. The sample evaluation form (Fig. 6-1) measures the nurse against the performance criteria described earlier in this chapter.

	Always	Usually	Sometimes	Rarely	Shows Improvement	Needs Improvement
A. PRIMARY NURSE ROLE:						
1. Selects and maintains two or more primary patients at all times	___	___	___	___	___	___
2. Identifies role to patients, physicians, family, and staff	___	___	___	___	___	___
3. Selects associate nurses	___	___	___	___	___	___
4. Initiates admission interview, History & Physical	___	___	___	___	___	___
5. Initiates and reflects changes on the Primary Nursing Care Plan	___	___	___	___	___	___
6. Reflects pertinent observations on Kardex	___	___	___	___	___	___
7. Records assessments and observations in chart	___	___	___	___	___	___
8. Maintains communication triangle	___	___	___	___	___	___
9. Maintains Buddy System	___	___	___	___	___	___
10. Initiates patient-centered conferences	___	___	___	___	___	___
11. Initiates discharge planning	___	___	___	___	___	___
12. Evaluates for home visits	___	___	___	___	___	___

Fig. 6-1. Staff evaluation form.

	Always	Usually	Sometimes	Rarely	Shows Improvement	Needs Improvement
B. ASSOCIATE NURSE ROLE:						
1. Accepts and/or selects role	___	___	___	___	___	___
2. Identifies role to patients, physicians, family, and staff	___	___	___	___	___	___
3. Continues care planned by Primary Nurse	___	___	___	___	___	___
4. Reflects changes on the Primary Nursing Care Plan	___	___	___	___	___	___
5. Reflects pertinent observations on Kardex	___	___	___	___	___	___
6. Records assessments and observations in chart	___	___	___	___	___	___
7. Maintains communication triangle in Primary Nurse's absence	___	___	___	___	___	___
8. Maintains Buddy System	___	___	___	___	___	___
9. Participates or initiates patient-centered conferences	___	___	___	___	___	___
10. Continues discharge planning	___	___	___	___	___	___
C. STAFF DEVELOPMENT:						
1. Defines/accepts unit objectives and performance criteria	___	___	___	___	___	___
2. Identifies own capabilities and limitations	___	___	___	___	___	___

Continued.

Fig. 6-1, cont'd. Staff evaluation form.

The nurse on this evaluation form is measured for both performance and attitude toward performance. For example, although the nurse may make independent decisions "rarely," the rating "shows improvement" is also checked. In this way the rating "rarely" does not sit as a failure for the nurse. Rather, the rating "shows improvement" indicates that an effort is being made by the nurse to

		Always	Usually	Sometimes	Rarely	Shows Improvement	Needs Improvement
3.	Accepts constructive criticism and makes appropriate changes	___	___	___	___	___	___
4.	Positively reinforces coworkers' capabilities	___	___	___	___	___	___
5.	Gives constructive criticism	___	___	___	___	___	___
6.	Promotes a cohesive work environment	___	___	___	___	___	___
7.	Promotes peer review	___	___	___	___	___	___
8.	Participates in decision making	___	___	___	___	___	___
9.	Identifies areas for expanded roles	___	___	___	___	___	___
10.	Identifies growth opportunities in shift rotation	___	___	___	___	___	___
11.	Attends staff meetings and workshops	___	___	___	___	___	___
12.	Attends community workshops	___	___	___	___	___	___

D. PROBLEM SOLVING:

1.	Considers a broad analysis of problems	___	___	___	___	___	___
2.	Considers multiple resources and sources of information	___	___	___	___	___	___

Fig. 6-1, cont'd. Staff evaluation form.

improve. A rating of "rarely," however, indicates more counseling is needed if "needs improvement" is also checked.

Counseling during the evaluation includes both feedback for the past six months and a comparison to previous evaluations. The staff nurse will understand more readily progress or lack of progress.

	Always	Usually	Sometimes	Rarely	Shows Improvement	Needs Improvement
3. Considers alternative interventions	___	___	___	___	___	___
4. Assigns priorities to problems and interventions	___	___	___	___	___	___
5. Reviews consequences of alternative interventions	___	___	___	___	___	___
6. Makes decisions based upon conclusions formulated from the above	___	___	___	___	___	___
7. Implements a plan for intervention	___	___	___	___	___	___
8. Evaluates results of the intervention as a basis for further growth and development	___	___	___	___	___	___

E. COMMENTS:

_____   _____
Staff Member   Head Nurse

Fig. 6-1, cont'd. Staff evaluation form.

An evaluation conference can be more meaningful when a dialogue occurs. This dialogue implies that the staff nurse and head nurse evaluate each other. The staff nurse also evaluates the assistant head nurse and unit in-service coordinator on a six-month basis. If the responsibility of unit leaders is to provide quality patient care standards and staff development, it is essential that they get

```
Head Nurse_____    Date_____
or
Assistant Head Nurse_____     By Whom_____
or
In-service Coordinator_____


A.  Attitude and Strengths


B.  Leadership (planning, leading, organizing, controlling)


C.  Resource Person (clinical, psysho-social, problem solving, etc.)


D.  Role Model (communication, professional, etc.)


E.  Staff Development (individual, group)


F.  Areas Needing Improvement


G.  How can you be helped more individually?


H.  Unit suggestions:


I.  Additional Comments:



Leader                          Evaluated by:
```

Fig. 6-2. Unit leadership evaluation form.

feedback from the staff regarding their attitudes and performance. The leadership evaluation form (Fig. 6-2) provides unit leaders insight and reinforcement for their roles as well as lists their problem areas requiring improvement.

In evaluating the assistant head nurse and in-service coordinator, the head nurse can draw from staff evaluations as well as from her own observations. The head nurse, by sharing staff evaluations of the unit leaders with the supervisor for the unit and with the director of nursing, helps to compile a more global evaluation of the unit itself.

Primary nursing care plans. In addition to serving as effective communication tools for continued individualized patient care, primary nursing care plans can be utilized as evaluation tools. As discussed in Chapter 3, the care plans describe in detail the twenty-four–hour plan for care and the nurse's assessment of the patient's situation. The head nurse and other staff members reviewing the care plan can obtain an accurate picture of the nurse's ability to assess a patient's physical and psychosocial well-being. Physician, staff, and patient feedback from daily patient rounds can serve as a comparison against the care plan. Finally, patient-centered conferences, in which the care plan is discussed, further highlight the nurse's assessment and problem-solving abilities.

Nursing audits. The nursing audit is a systematized approach for evaluating the quality of care provided and further asserts nursing responsibility and authority for measurement of the quality of nursing care given. Improvements will be made then on the basis of audit findings. Phaneuf[6] suggests that to facilitate the urgently needed changes in health care and delivery systems, more nursing emphasis on data and on explicit judgments are needed. A more disciplined and intellectual nursing approach to quality appraisal of care needs to be instituted.

Nursing audits proposed at the unit level become a simplified form of hospital audits. Audits can promote evaluation and improvement of standards of quality care and of staff performance. Peer review, an outgrowth of nursing audits, can stimulate a constructive form of assessment in which staff members in cooperation with the head nurse evaluate and stimulate improvements toward quality patient care.

On a primary nursing unit, daily nursing audits of each shift routinely evaluate quality standards of care and staff performance. Appraisal is expected by the staff, as are improvements in care and performance when necessary.

After a unit audit committee is established, the chairman for this committee or her replacement can schedule nurses on the unit to act as auditors. The schedules, which should give at least a week's advance notice, can be posted and may include unit leaders. However, unit leaders should generally be used in resource capacities for the auditor. The unit audit committee is initiated to set standards for care involving unit personnel, physicians, and supervisors. The hospital audit committee can act as a resource for the unit committee. Together they can develop audit forms as guidelines for evaluating quality care standards.

Patients can be selected at random by the auditor from a list of patients not previously audited. Primary nurses are accountable for meeting with the auditor, although associate nurses can serve as a replacement. Audit feedback to the head nurse is expected to be automatic, as is a review of audit findings during staff meetings. Documentation of audit data can be maintained by the in-service coordinator and kept available for staff.

Patient supervision and safety, medical diagnosis and rationale for care, observations of symptoms and reactions, promotion of physical and emotional health by direction and teaching, and supervision of other health personnel constitute the areas that are evaluated on the unit audit. Primary nurses, who are accountable for total patient care, continuance of care, and teaching, are stimulated to learn, evaluate, and amend their approaches to care by nursing audits.

More specifically, the auditor and primary nurse examine the complete medical chart and, if possible, interview the patient to obtain his perceptions of his care. Together they confirm that the physician's orders are accurately reflected on the Kardex and that they have been executed and charted properly. The primary nurse discusses the medical diagnosis and rationale for care. Together they confirm that the rationale is reflected on the primary nursing care plan and that corresponding documentation occurs in the nurse's notes. They confirm also that teaching areas are reflected in the care plan and that corresponding documentation is evident. Intervention by and supervision of other hospital personnel in the patient's care is discussed by the primary nurse and evaluated by the auditor.

Each of these categories is then delineated to give the auditor specific guidelines and corresponding number values. As in most nursing audits, a word judgment of quality can be assigned to a number (for example, excellent = 200). Follow through by the auditor and primary nurse is expected for audits that produce results less than excellent. Appropriate improvements and confirmation of those improvements are evaluated again at a set time decided by the audit committee.

The primary nurse then communicates the audit results to associate nurses, buddies, and other staff members involved in the patient's care. Patient safety, nurse development, and a holistic approach to patient care by the nursing staff can be enhanced by unit nursing audits.

Formal research. Research tools can be used not only to evaluate change but also as a stimulus for change. Although the purpose of research is to measure change, a commensurate advantage is that it provides stimulation as a result of the introduction of questionnaires. Administration of questionnaires can facilitate the progress toward change because staff expect that their progress will be measured. Our research is described in Chapters 7 to 10.

Staff meetings and staff workshops. Weekly staff meetings promote good interstaff communication and can include hospital and unit activities, policies, and plans. They can also provide a formalized time for staff to evaluate their progress and to problem solve as a group. If specific areas are to be discussed or evaluated, the head nurse can post the topics in advance so that staff will come prepared to discuss them. Staff meetings as well as staff workshops can be documented for the review of the entire staff.

Monthly staff workshops held off the unit can also provide the staff formalized time and a more relaxed atmosphere than that of staff meetings for evaluation and collective decision-making and problem-solving activities. Projects can be evaluated, and new projects can be proposed and outlined in more detail with a greater number of staff present.

SUMMARY

The processes of change necessary to implement primary nursing are many and include several phases that advance the idea and theory of primary nursing to a sustained operating system of care. Implementing primary nursing starts with the perception of a need for change in the existing nursing care modality. Administrators, physicians, and nurses, especially the director of nursing, all play key roles in establishing and maintaining a commitment to change. Nursing personnel will undergo redefinition of their roles, and this redefining process will help to carve the foundation for primary nursing. By the time actual implementation occurs, the head nurse, staff, and nursing administration have a detailed schedule of expected events, which helps them realize even little successes. Finally, the change that has occurred must be maintained and evaluated. Performance criteria, staff evaluations, primary nursing care plans, nursing audits, staff meetings and workshops, and formal research require staff to measure their progress against their goals. These processes of evaluation in turn stimulate further change to occur. Primary nursing is grounded in a cyclical pursuit toward achieving its objectives when change is a collaborative and cooperative endeavor that includes staff as well as key organization administrators.

REFERENCES

1. Gilbert, Albert E.: Managing change in the hospital, Hospital Topics **47:**40-41, 1969.
2. Bennis, W. G.: Changing organizations, New York, 1966, McGraw-Hill Book Co., Inc.
3. Sheehan, Dorothy: The director's defection, American Journal of Nursing **73:**485-490, 1973.
4. Manthey, Marie: Primary care is alive and well in the hospital, American Journal of Nursing **73:**83-87, 1973.
5. Bevis, E. O.: Curriculum change, St. Louis, 1973, The C. V. Mosby Co., p. 248.
6. Phaneuf, Maria C.: The nursing audit, New York, 1972, Meredith Corporation.

SUGGESTED READINGS

Bennis, W. G., Benne, K. D., and Chin, R.: The planning of change, New York, 1961, Holt, Rinehart & Winston, Inc.
Luft, J.: Group processes, Palo Alto, Calif., 1966, National Press.
Rubin, C. F., Rinaldi, L. A., and Dietz, R. R.: Nursing audit—nurses evaluating nursing, American Journal of Nursing **72:**916-922, 1972.
Seiler, J. A.: Systems analysis in organizational behavior, Homewood, Ill., 1967, Dorsey Press, Inc.

III

EFFECTS OF PRIMARY NURSING

chapter 7

OUTCOMES FOR THE PATIENT

Verbally or nonverbally the patient informs his physician, family, friends, fellow patients, and (at best) the nurse who is in direct charge of his care just what he thinks of the nursing care he is getting. If several nurses are attending to his needs, the chances that he will trust one nurse well enough or will be given enough of the nurse's time to elaborate his opinions of his care are extremely small.[1] The opportunities provided to patients to put their comments in writing are even more infrequent. However, patients do have opinions about nurses and nursing care, and studies have shown that these opinions can be categorized. According to Price,[2] patients generally comment on the following:

1. Promptness of nurses
2. Friendliness of nurses
3. Their confidence in nurses' abilities
4. Nurses' consideration of patients' likes and dislikes with respect to their care
5. Efficiency of the nursing staff in providing care
6. Frequency that nurses check on them
7. Nurses' acceptance and understanding of them

In summary, patients' reactions to nursing care are often global and reflect their attitudes about many aspects of patient involvement in the hospital. However, when patients are asked to reflect on their nursing care in particular, they frequently respond in terms of several consistent criteria. These criteria reflect patients' needs for a secure environment in which their uniqueness is perceived, understood, and, hopefully, integrated in the planning, execution, and evaluation of their care.

Questionnaires distributed to patients about their care received under a primary nursing care delivery system contained these and other categories. Patients responded openly and freely to requests for their perceptions and attitudes.

THE STUDY

To compare the perceptions of patients on primary nuring units with the perceptions of patients on other nursing units, we developed questionnaires to be administered to samples of patients on each kind of unit. A study of two different hospitals gave us a total sample of 360 patients—120 patients from primary nursing units, 120 patients from team nursing units, sixty from functional nursing care units and sixty from case method units. This sample was further broken down to conduct specific analyses of patient groups (for example, comparing sixty patients before and after implementation of primary nursing on the units and comparing matched samples, according to a certain time period, of patients on primary, team, case, and functional nursing units).

With the aid of research assistants, we used a combination of procedures to gain patients' responses to the questions. Our chief approach was to leave a questionnaire with each patient to be completed without the presence of the researcher. Only when patients were too sick to read or unable to write their responses did the researcher record patients' responses on the questionnaire.

Patients' responses to the questionnaires, which were designed to tap their level of satisfaction with nursing care and their impressions of the nature of their care, pointed out some important features of primary nursing care.

PREDICTIONS ABOUT EFFECTS OF PRIMARY NURSING ON PATIENTS

Prior to collecting data from patients, some assumptions and propositions about the outcome of primary nursing were formulated. These propositions were reconstructed as hypotheses and guided the collection of data. A chief assumption of the study was that primary nursing has at least six distinct organizational outcomes, which have an indirect, if not direct, effect on the patient's perception of his care. These outcomes are as follows:

1. Personalized delivery of patient care, including increased accessibility of the nurse to the patient and his family
2. Individualized implementation of patient care
3. Patient-cooperative planning and implementation of his care with his primary nurse
4. A rational basis for delivery of nursing care (that is, the nurse who knows the most about the patient is responsible for his care and held accountable)
5. Increased accountability of the nurse for total comprehensive patient care
6. Increased continuity and coordination of patient care

In our study it was assumed that primary nursing would be unhampered by the intervention of multiple nursing personnel, thus making nursing the delivery of direct nursing care from one (primary) nurse to the patient. The nurse would treat the patient as a unique being, distinguished from a class or collection of patients. We visualized primary nursing as not only noticing the individuality of patients but also treating the distinctness and complexity of patients as individuals. Nurses in this one-to-one relationship with patients could involve patients in the assessment, planning, implementation, and evaluation of their nursing care. Because nurses would be assigned total care for their patients, nurses knowing the most about patients and their families would give them care and thus would be held accountable for the patients' reaction to nursing interventions. Their responsibility for total patient comprehensive care would be enhanced by their continuous involvement in every aspect of patient interest—whether financial, spiritual, physical, or emotional. Nurses' ability to promote continuity would be considerably heightened, since they would be in close contact with the patient throughout his hospitalization, and fewer nursing personnel would intercede to complicate the achievement of both long- and short-term nursing goals.

COMPARISON OF PATIENTS' PERCEPTIONS ON PRIMARY NURSING, CASE METHOD, FUNCTIONAL NURSING, AND TEAM NURSING UNITS

An initial phase of the study was to compare the perceptions of primary patients with those of patients on other units. Questionnaires were administered in two hospitals at different times to sets of patients on case method, functional, primary, and team nursing units. Responses of sixty patients on primary nursing units were compared with those of 120 patients on other types of units collected in the same time period.

Individualized and personalized patient care. Patients on all units were asked to list those things they liked about their nursing care and the problems they saw.

As predicted a genuine *concern for the individual patient* and *personalized approach* to his care were the most frequently mentioned characteristics of the primary nursing care units by patients on these units (Tables 7-1, 4, and 7-2, 2). Patients on primary nursing care units not only mentioned these characteristics frequently in describing their nursing care but, in addition, mentioned it most frequently as having the greatest importance to them. Clearly these patients believed that they had received personalized attention and that the nurses truly regarded "the patient as a person."

The second most frequently mentioned group of characteristics were the at-

Table 7-1. What patients liked best about their nursing care

| | Frequency mentioned (%/rank) | | | |
| | Primary nursing units (N = 60) | Case method nursing units (N = 30) | Team nursing units (N = 60) | Functional nursing units (N = 30) |
Category of response				
1 Pleasantness of nurse	25%/no. 2	35%/no. 2	36%/no. 1	20%/no. 2
2 Promptness of nurse	17%/no. 3	10%/no. 3	23%/no. 2	39%/no. 1
3 Nurse's ability	3%/no. 5	4%/no. 5	12.5%/no. 4	20%/no. 3
4 Nurse's consideration of patient individuality	51%/no. 1	45%/no. 1	21.5%/no. 3	15%/no. 4
5 Physical care considerations (e.g., back rubs)	4%/no. 4	6%/no. 4	7%/no. 5	6%/no. 5

Table 7-2. Patients' perceptions of their nurses and nursing care

	Percentage of patients agreeing or strongly agreeing			
Patients' views of nurse's behavior and attitudes	Primary nursing units (N = 60)	Case method units (N = 30)	Team nursing units (N = 60)	Functional nursing units (N = 30)
1 Nurse gives emotional support frequently	85%	80%	60%	63%
2 Nurse treats patients like special human beings	95%	93%	51%	47%
3 Nurse is too concerned with others' perceptions and not with what patient's think they need	0	0	20%	25%
4 Finishing on time is more important to nurse than good care	0	0	15%	17%
5 Nurse spends more time with patient than with other tasks	28%	15%	0	10%

titudes of individual nurses; that is, they were "kind," "considerate," "helpful," "cheerful," and "pleasant." Positive actions of nurses such as responding to requests promptly, carrying out physicians' orders effectively, offering the opportunity for back rubs, and others, although mentioned as important and present on the unit, took a back seat to the importance of the individualized care. One patient on a primary nursing care unit succinctly described it in his answer to the question, "What problems with your nursing care have you identified?" He said, "I can identify no problem—if there has been any, it runs along the line of how can so many terrific people maintain such a continuing interest in *me*?"[3]

To indicate how differently she perceived nursing on primary nursing units, one patient recounted the following experience that she had in another hospital—an experience that was obviously despairing:

> . . . an old lady in an adjacent bed had a postop tube inserted through her nose into her stomach. When she rang for a nurse, she was forced to talk loud enough for the speaker over her bed to pick it up. In other words, she was treated no differently from a relatively well patient. Individual treatment was completely lacking. Not so with primary nursing.

Patients on primary nursing units did believe they were being treated as unique persons with distinct individual differences.

Another patient explained:

> In other hospitalizations I had been made to feel I was not a person, just a body attached to an arm band and a chart, necessitating constant check to them (the armband and the chart) to see that I was getting the correct medication or treatment at the convenience of the staff. The nurses, although capable, always seemed rushed,

harrassed, and often resentful of some higher authority. The general attitude was that the personnel were working at a job, which, regardless of the patient's desires or previous personal habits, had to be altered to fit "the system." With my primary nurse I felt that she would not be too rushed to be with me when and if I needed her, yet I would not be disturbed if I wanted to be alone.

These patients' comments were in direct contrast with comments of patients who did not have primary nurses.

Whereas personalized and individualized attention was mentioned frequently as the aspect of their care that patients on primary nursing units liked most, this feature clearly took a far less conspicuous role in patients' descriptions of the nursing care that they were receiving on team and functional nursing units.*

Pleasantness and patience of nurses in general, as well as promptness and attention to physical aspects of care were more frequently on the minds of patients on team and functional nursing units when they described their care (Table 7-1). With the exception of one unit, patients found nurses to be lacking in the sincere concern for the individual patient shown by nurses on primary nursing units. According to one patient on a team nursing unit: "They act like they could care less instead of understand and be helpful." Another patient on another unit replied: "Some of the nurses are much too impersonal and machinelike. They made me feel more like an object than a human being." Another patient, verifying the extreme that the patient may interpret his nurses' indifference and insensitivity to his unique needs, replied: "You don't ask nurses to come in too much as they will get mean and not take care of you."

Patients' sense of efficacy and security regarding their nursing care. It was hypothesized that primary nursing, since it is a system of individualized and personalized patient care, would have a significant effect on the patient's sense of efficacy and security in the hospital. Primary nursing promises increased relevancy of care to the patient, reinforced by the continuous one-to-one relationship between nurse and patient. Patients would be more likely to participate in their own care. Patients' fears and anxiety would be low because of their increased involvement in their own care, because of the greater continuity in their nursing care, and because the nurse who knows the most about the patient is responsible for his care and accountable for the outcomes of this care.

In summary, it was anticipated that primary nursing would foster a socioemotional climate for the patient that would give him a sense of power and trust about what would happen to him.

Patients were asked to give their opinions on ten descriptive statements about their nurses and their nursing care. Patients rated their nurses by indicating whether they strongly agreed, agreed, felt neutral, disagreed, or strongly disagreed with the statements.

---

*Team nursing practiced on the other units involved shared responsibility among nurses for planning, implementing, and evaluating each patient's care. Continuity of any *one* nurse-patient relationship was rarely obtained or viewed as essential by nurses.

It was predicted that patients on the primary nursing units would have a greater sense of efficacy about their care, a greater sense that nurses cared about them, and a greater sense that the care given them was the best and of the highest priority to the nurse.

Primary nurses were especially perceived by patients to treat patients' opinions with high regard (Table 7-2, 3). Patients rated primary nurses as highly interested in what patients thought they needed. Primary nurses were seen to be more concerned with patients' getting the best care possible than with all the work getting done (Table 7-2, 4). One patient aptly described what he viewed as the main interest of the primary nurse:

> The nurse directs her time and effort on the basis of patient need, not on the basis that all beds must be made up in waltz time by midmorning. Housekeeping chores assume a lower priority, but this doesn't mean they don't get done. They do get done but only after the nurse has satisfied her personal patient care priority program.

Finally, primary nurses were perceived to spend a great deal of time at the patient's bedside (Table 7-2, 5). How the priority of the nurse was interpreted by the patient in light of his needs for security is evident from the following responses. One patient explained:

> There was never any time that I did not feel secure in the knowledge that the staff was, so to speak, "on top of it," and, should an emergency arise, it would be handled promptly, efficiently, and with as little stress projected to the patient as possible.

Another patient clearly stated how he thought his situation differed from that which might occur with team nursing:

> The patient is made to feel that there is interest in him and the primary nurse is familiar with his case. She is competent and enthusiastic about her work. Schedules are accommodated to the patient's needs and desires. In another hospital, patient care was the responsibility of a team—no one member of which knew the whole story or gave a damn. The work appeared to be a means to an end rather than the end itself.

Although a direct relationship seemed to exist between patients' perceptions of how they were treated and their perceptions of their security in the hospital setting of nursing, there were many exceptions. Patient responses indicated that they can feel secure about their nursing care and at the same time feel that they are treated systematically, as objects rather than as unique persons.

On cardiac care units where functional nursing was practiced, for example, the nurse was perceived by the patient to spend a great amount of time at the bedside giving "expert" care; but, at the same time, patients still felt that the nurse cared less about treating them as special persons. More often than primary nursing patients, these patients thought that they were treated like objects by the nurse and that they had little or no influence on how their care was delivered.

On team and functional nursing units patients' sense of efficacy and security was much lower than that of patients on either primary nursing or case method units. Patients were more likely to view nurses as more concerned with getting their work done on time than with making sure that patients received the best possible care.

In addition, patients did not believe that nurses considered their opinions important. They thought nurses were more concerned with others' opinions (such as physicians) and were not interested enough in what the patients thought they needed in the hospital.

In summary, when patients perceived their care as highly individualized and personalized, they were more likely to feel secure with their care and to feel as if they had some influence on how their care was delivered. However, safe and efficient care did not necessarily give them a sense of efficacy or a sense of being treated as special persons. The latter was found to be especially true with patients on specialty units, in which the functional method was the chief modality for nursing care delivery.

Patients' satisfaction and adjustment to hospitalization. Because significant attitude differences were noted in patients with primary nurses, it was anticipated that their overall satisfaction with their nursing care and adjustment to hospitalization and their illness might vary from that of patients who did not experience primary nursing.

Patients' level of satisfaction, numbers of complaints, and incidences of verbalization and working through emotional reactions to hospilization and illness were recorded, and their ability to follow prescribed treatment regimens was also noted.

Primary nursing care patients' satisfaction with their care was exceptional as noted from the consistent and large amount of feedback, which included letters that went to individual nurses as well as to hospital administrators. Several patients made donations to one primary nursing care unit, having recognized its special character and wanting to contribute to the primary nursing endeavor. Patients willingly volunteered (without prompting) comments of satisfaction. Approximately 65 percent of the patients on primary nursing units, compared with 37 percent on team nursing units, 48 percent on functional nursing units, and 40 percent on case method units explained in a formal questionnaire that they were extremely satisfied with their nursing care (Table 7-3).

The lack of complaints from primary nursing care patients and their families is equally impressive. Two strong indicators that patients' needs are being met by these primary nurses are (1) the minimum use of lights to beckon nurses to the rooms and (2) the minimum incidents of family members coming to the central desk as concerned spokesmen for patients. Patients on primary nursing units seemed to use the call button and/or rely on family members to get them what they needed less frequently than did patients on floors where team nursing was operant.

Patients with primary nurses were also known to follow through on physicians' prescribed treatment regimens. In part, this can be attributed to the consistent surveillance of the primary nurse, as well as to the fact that follow-up visits in the

Table 7-3. Patients' satisfaction with their nursing care

Level of satisfaction	Primary nursing units (N = 60)	Case method units (N = 30)	Team nursing units (N = 60)	Functional nursing units (N = 30)
Extremely satisfied	65%	40%	37%	48%
Very satisfied	32%	40%	41%	21%
Moderately satisfied	3%	15%	10%	12%
Slightly satisfied	0	5%	11%	9%
Not at all satisfied	0	0	1%	10%

home were a facet of some primary nursing care units. However, the importance of the patient's attitude that his care is "tailored" to him and therefore more relevant cannot be denied as sufficient reason for the patient to follow through on his physician's orders.

We are presently collecting data on the rehospitalization rate of primary nursing care patients as compared to patients without primary nurses. We have already estimated that the rehospitalization rate of primary patients is lower; however, we need further empirical data to substantiate our findings to date.

The majority of patients working through problems with their nurses about their illnesses and hospitalization is probably more accurately portrayed in kind than in number. More primary nursing patients entered into important self-disclosures and worked through conflicts and anxieties than did other patients. This is attributed not so much to personality characteristics of nurses and patients or to the severity of the illness as to the opportunities for nurses and patients to develop trusting relationships, in which patients are sure that their nurses know and care about them. Primary nursing facilitates the formation of cohesive one-to-one relationship between nurse and patient.

COMPARISON OF PATIENTS' PERCEPTIONS BEFORE AND AFTER IMPLEMENTATION OF PRIMARY NURSING

As indicated earlier, the two essential strategies to our study of primary nursing were as follows: to compare patients on primary nursing units with those on other nursing units (see previous section for results of this part of the study) and to compare patients on a unit before and after the implementation of primary nursing. With this tactic, any peculiarities of nurses on the unit or physical outlay of the unit could be controlled. This second type of comparison could provide more data about the results of implementing primary nursing.

The findings strongly substantiated those results mentioned thus far and are as follows. First, patients on the unit before and after primary nursing differed in their attitudes about what was the most desirable aspect of their care. After the implementation of primary nursing, patients mentioned individual concern for

Table 7-4. What patients liked best about their care before and after
primary nursing

	Frequency mentioned (%/rank)	
Category of response	Before (N = 60)	After (N = 60)
1 Pleasantness of nurse	42.9%/no. 1	20%/no. 2
2 Promptness of nurse	28.6%/no. 2	16%/no. 3
3 Nurse's ability	4.2%/no. 3	0%/no. 5
4 Nurse's consideration of patient individuality	28.6%/no. 2	44%/no. 1
5 Physical care considerations (e.g., back rubs)	0%/no. 4	4%/no. 4

Table 7-5. Patients' perceptions of their nurses and nursing care before
and after primary nursing implementation

	Percentage of patients agreeing or strongly agreeing	
Patients' view of nurse's behavior and attitudes	Before (N = 60)	After (N = 60)
1 Nurse gives emotional support frequently	35%	75%
2 Nurse treats patients like special human beings	30%	95%
3 Finishing on time is more important to nurse than giving good care	15%	0
4 Nurse spends more time with patient than with other tasks	5%	15%
5 Nurse is too concerned with others' perceptions and not with what patient's think they need	15%	0

the patient more frequently and pleasantness and promptness less frequently
Table 7-4 contains a detailed comparison of patient's perceptions before and after
the implementation of primary nursing.

Second, patients thought that they became a higher priority to the nurse after
the implementation of primary nursing. They perceived that their care was more
geared toward their individual uniqueness as special people in need of emotional
support. After the conversion of the unit to primary nursing, patients were more
likely to view the nurse as concerned with giving them the best possible care (not
just with getting the job done on time) and interested in what they themselves
thought they needed as patients (Table 7-5).

Table 7-6. Patients' satisfaction before and after implementation of primary nursing

Level of satisfaction	Before (N = 60)	After (N = 60)
Extremely satisfied	29%	64%
Very satisfied	58%	24%
Moderately satisfied	0	12%
Slightly satisfied	0	0
Not at all satisfied	13%	0

The final comparison of the general satisfaction of patients before and after the implementation of primary nursing also substantiated our earlier findings. After the implementation of primary nursing, more patients said that they were either extremely or very satisfied with their nursing care; 64 percent of the patients were extremely satisfied with their nursing care after implementation of primary nursing, compared to 29 percent before implementation of primary nursing on the units (Table 7-6).

SUMMARY

From the patient's point of view, primary nursing is a personalized and individualized system of meeting his nursing care needs. Nurses' promptness, general friendliness, and efficiency take a backseat in the minds of primary nursing patients to the nurses' ability to know and treat patients as individuals. The findings indicate that not only did primary nursing patients have different expectations of their nursing care, but their general sense of security and trust behaviors also differed. Patients cooperated more and complained less about their care. Their general sense of security and confidence in the efficacy and competence of their nurses freed them from the typical fears of hospitalization that are experienced by all patients, concerning whether their nurses would or could take care of them if they really needed them.

The study imparted a distinct impression that primary nursing patients thought they could and should evaluate their nurses and physicians, in addition to expressing themselves about the overall environment of the unit. With their enhanced sense of influence, patients would no longer tolerate abuse or humiliation and they would not allow their chief guardian, their primary nurse, to be humiliated or belittled.

Primary nursing does more than reflect the future of nursing care—a future in which patients emerge as unique individuals who demand a voice in how their nursing care is delivered and what the focus of that care should be. Primary nursing mirrors the past. As one patient explained: "It brought to mind the 'old days of nursing care' when nurses were nursing, and you were treated as an individual with the staff having the time and the trained personnel to know their patients and anticipate their needs."

REFERENCES

1. Marram, G.: Patients' evaluation of their care: importance to the nurse, Nursing Outlook **21:**322-325, May, 1973.
2. Price, E.: Staffing for patient care, New York, 1970, Springer Publishing Co., Inc., p. 146.
3. Marram, G.: Innovation on Four Tower West—what happened? American Journal of Nursing **73:**814-817, 1973.

SUGGESTED READINGS

Abdellah, F. G., Martin A., Belord, I. L., and Matheney, R. V.: Patient-centered approaches to nursing, New York, 1961, The Macmillan Co.

Allen, E. M.: Information viewed most helpful to patients undergoing three selected diagnostic procedures, American Nurses Association Clinical Conferences, 1969.

Blau, P. M.: Orientation toward clients in a public welfare agency. In Zauk, M., and Mayer, N., editors: Social welfare institutions, New York, 1965, John Wiley & Sons, Inc.

Deutsch, E. B.: A stereotype—or an individual, Nursing Outlook **19:**106-110, Feb., 1971.

Kramer, M.: Standard 4—nursing care plans—power to the patient, Journal of Nursing Administration, pp. 29-34, Sept.-Oct., 1972.

Manthey, M., Ciske, K., Robertson, P., and Harris, I.: Primary nursing, Nursing Forum **9:**65-83, 1970.

Marram, G.: Patients' evaluations of nursing performance, Nursing Research **22:**153-157, March-April, 1973.

Nehring, V., and Geach, B.: Patients' evaluation of their care: why they don't complain, Nursing Outlook **21:**317-322, May, 1973.

Schmidt, J.: Availability—a concept of nursing practice, American Journal of Nursing **72:**1086-1090, 1972.

chapter 8

EFFECTS ON THE NURSING PERSONNEL

It is not by accident that primary nursing has sprung up in a number of acute care agencies across the country. As noted in earlier chapters, the timing is right. Several trends in the health care delivery system make primary nursing a logical outgrowth of the evolution of nursing care modalities. The need for better continuity and better coordination of nursing care and greater accountability to the patient for his nursing care are only a few factors stimulating hospitals to experiment with primary nursing care.

Surely the use and misuse of professional nurses in the hospital has supported the trend toward more independent, accountable nursing care. Leininger, Little, and Carnevali[1] suggest that any kind of primary care should be a great deal more satisfying to professional nurses. They claim that it should help professional nurses use their skills and broad nursing educational background more fully. Heretofore professional nurses, especially those graduating from baccalaureate programs, were poorly used by the hospital system of nursing. Compared to team or functional nursing, primary nursing should do a better job of helping nurses realize their potential with the individual patient and his family.

As noted in Chapter 3, there is a concerted effort on the part of nursing administrators of hospitals to consider alternatives to team and functional nursing. Experimental units are being erected in several institutions to assess new modalities in nursing, including primex, primary care, and primary nursing. Although these units are arising because of deliberate planning by nursing administrators, decisions to implement primary nursing are not the result of administrative efforts alone. In several settings including agencies, hospitals, and others, highly professional and change-oriented head nurses, supervisors, and staff nurse groups who are strongly committed to experimentation have encouraged the director of nurses to facilitate the development of experimental units. As the in-service instructor and clinical nursing coordinator of the primary nursing pediatric unit at one university medical center so aptly described the situation there: "Lack of direct patient care and fragmentation of care caused the nursing staff themselves to think and work toward changing the system." Nurses at the unit level had much to gain by these changes. Organizing nursing tasks so that the entire care of one patient is the responsibility of a single nurse not only addresses desires of nurses to give "idealized" patient care but also promises them more autonomy and recognition as staff nurses.

THE STUDY

For the evaluation of the effects of primary nursing on registered nurses and licensed vocational nurses, several sources of data were available. Informal comments of nurses on the primary nursing units were monitored. Detailed questionnaires were used to measure nurses' attitudes about the way their work was organized. Their value orientations as well as their overall satisfaction with their work on the primary nursing care units were compared with those of nurses on other nursing modality units. In addition, periodic formal evaluations of nurses' performance on the primary care units were at our disposal.

The formal questionnaire, more than any other instrument used, gave empirical data about differences between primary nurses and nurses not practicing primary nursing. Because data collected were from nurses practicing team nursing, functional nursing, the case method approach, and primary nursing, the findings presented here gain added validity. A comparison of team, functional, and case method nursing units with primary nursing units demonstrates how groups of nurses on primary units differed from groups of nurses on other kinds of units. Our time-sequence data, which compares nurses before and after implementation of primary nursing, gives information about changes in nurses with the new modality of nursing care.

Since it forms the basis for later discussion, a more specific explanation of the administration of the formal questionnaire to nurses is warranted, describing the various steps that are necessary to gain reliable evidence about primary nursing.

Essentially two patterns of data collection were utilized: (1) intra-unit measurements, in which nurses were compared with themselves before and after the implementation of primary nursing and (2) cross-unit comparison, in which nurses on primary nursing units were compared with nurses on other units. The formal questionaire was the same for both measurements, since it was necessary to establish a uniform tool. The formal questionnaire was used to compare forty-five primary nurses before and after implementation of primary nursing in two different hospitals and to compare forty-five primary nurses with sixty-five nurses practicing team, functional, or case method nursing.

Controls were exerted to make sure that what was being measured on the primary care units was more the result of primary nursing than a result of any other strong significant factor.

Essentially one approach was used to gain nurses' responses to the formal questionnaires. Nurses were given the questionnaires to fill out at their leisure, returning them to an envelope addressed to one of us (G.D.M.) who would pick them up on the respective units. Nurses were told that their responses would be kept secret and that their participation (or lack of it) would not be held against them in any way. Surprisingly enough, all but a few nurses participated in the study.

Nurses' responses to these questionnaires, which were designed to tap their level of satisfaction with the way their work was organized and their professional value orientation pointed out some important effects that primary nursing has on nursing staff. These outcomes will be discussed as they relate to our prediction regarding the effects of primary nursing on nurses.

PREDICTIONS ABOUT EFFECTS OF ORGANIZATIONAL FEATURES OF PRIMARY NURSING ON NURSES

It was predicted that primary nursing, like any other organized form of nursing care delivery, would have a great impact on the work of nurses and also on the involvement of nurses with their patients and their nursing tasks. This assumption was allowed to remain unchallenged. It was also anticipated that the six key organizational features of primary nursing discussed in Chapter 7 (p. 126) would have a definite impact on nurses.

The aspect of individualized and personalized care was predicted to affect the nurse in a number of ways. First, it was believed that in giving more individualized care, nurses would gain awareness of what they could do as individual change agents. Subscribing to patients as unique individuals would stimulate staff members to view themselves as distinct persons worth acknowledgment and development. This reinforcement of self-worth was believed to be visible in two ways —nurses asserting themselves more frequently and nurses expressing their overall satisfaction with their job, their motivation to stay in nursing, and their respect for nursing as a profession.

The more personalized the care that nurses could give, the greater opportunities they would have to alert to what the patient needed, given his unique sociopsychological framework. The more frequently that nurses could be successful and get feedback that they were successful, the greater their feelings of accomplishment with patients and efficacy as nurses would be. Again, this would result in greater satisfaction with their job and motivation to work as nurses.

In addition, the fact the primary nursing was a more rational basis for delivery of nursing care (that is, the most knowledgeable nurse gives the care) would also affect nurses. This rational basis for care would contribute not only to the greater efficacy of nurses and satisfaction with their performance but would also give them a sense of pride that they were participating in "idealized" patient care and administering high-quality nursing care.*

The kind of joint endeavor fostered between nurses and patients with primary nursing was anticipated to change nurses' attitudes about patients, as well as nurses' relationships with professional colleagues. The one-to-one, patient-nurse relationship was predicted to increase the number of times that the nurse consid-

---

*High-quality nursing care is viewed here as comprehensive nursing care in which the whole patient and his family are assessed, planned for, acted on, and evaluated for further intervention. Nurses use a problem-solving approach, secure continuity for their patients, and involve the patient and his family in planning the care given.

ered the patient's views. Patients and nurses would more likely be partners in patient care. Eliminating "middle-men" staff persons would also foster a direct colleague relationship among individual nurses and physicians and other professionals.

Increased equality among nursing staff could also be an outcome. Nurses might view other nurses as colleagues and not as "the nurse *above* me" or "the nurse *below* me." The status hierarchy accompanying team nursing would virtually be eliminated. Values about patient care would be rewarded more frequently than values about "directing other nurses."

This change in nursing hierarchy might be most noticeable in the treatment of licensed vocational nurses after their conversion to primary nursing roles. Thus it was predicted that L.V.N.s would make the biggest changes in terms of professional value orientation, satisfaction with their job, and perceptions of their self-worth in the new system.

Increased accountability for total patient care as well as greater continuity of nursing care should affect all primary nurses in many ways. It was believed that the added responsibility in the primary nursing role would result in only those nurses with confidence in themselves as nurses remaining in the new system.

Those nurses who fear total responsibility for patient care or who formerly took shelter in the supervision by their team leader would not choose the primary nursing system. Also, those nurses who, for whatever reason, avoid intensive and follow-up involvement with their patients would choose to go to other units. The nurses who stay on the primary nursing units should experience a better fit between their ideal image of nursing and what they were required to do on the job. Therefore the satisfaction of those nurses who remain should be high.

COMPARISON OF NURSES' RESPONSES ON PRIMARY NURSING AND TEAM, CASE METHOD, AND FUNCTIONAL NURSING UNITS

An initial phase of this study was to compare the perceptions of primary nurses with those of nurses on other kinds of nursing units in different hospitals. One important variable was the idealism of nurses at the start, which was defined as how recently the nurse had graduated from a nursing program and was controlled in the following manner. Primary nurses who were new graduates were not only compared with team nurses but also with other new graduates throughout the hospital. Responses of forty-five nurses on primary nursing units were compared with those of twenty-four nurses on team nursing units, twenty-five on case method units, and sixteen on functional nursing units.

Job satisfaction of nurses. As expected, those nurses practicing primary nursing had the highest rate of satisfaction with the way their work was organized.

When nurses were asked to record their satisfaction with the way their work was organized on their units (that is, whether extremely, very, moderately, slightly, or not at all satisfied), the following results were obtained: primary nurses were highest in job satisfaction; 90 percent of these nurses compared with

70 percent on case method units, 52 percent on team nursing units, and 43 percent on functional nursing units revealed that they were very or extremely satisfied.*

Table 8-1 is an account of how nurses' satisfaction differed on primary and other nursing units. Note that the highest percentage of responses for primary nurses fall in the very satisfied category, whereas team and functional nurses responses are more likely to fall in the category of moderately satisfied. The especially high satisfaction of nurses on primary nursing units can certainly be attributed in part to the large amount of positive feedback that they receive from their primary nursing patients, patients' families, physicians, and other nurses about their nursing care. The facts that they operate in a one-to-one relationship with patients, thus having more frequent opportunities for feedback, and that their efficacy is more visible to them are certainly factors fostering their job satisfaction. Most nurses reported that they liked primary nursing especially because it gave them consistent, in-depth involvement with a small number of patients and their families. Their relationships with patients had improved and become more meaningful. Perhaps the most significant factor about this change in the organization of their work, which also gave them great satisfaction, was that nurses were knowledgeable about a few patients as opposed to knowing a little about a lot of patients. In addition, the knowledge that they were contributing to nursing by validating a new approach gave them a great sense of pride and sense of accomplishment.

The high morale and motivation of primary nurses were perceived by patients, physicians, and administrators. Patients frequently commented that primary nurses were dedicated, proud, and happy to be nurses. Their strong sense of personal contribution to the cause of improved patient care was evident. The overall effect on the unit was that it became a more pleasant place for everybody, health personnel and patients.

Several hospitals reported that they were operating primary nursing units and that their staff did not want to go back to team nursing. The physicians and administrators shared this enthusiasm and satisfaction for the most part. (A more detailed account of their reactions is contained in Chapter 9.) Also, nurses were getting a better idea of how they could influence the recovery of their patients and did not want to lose the tremendous satisfaction and sense of efficacy that they had in planning, implementing, and evaluating total patient care.

---

* It is important when evaluating the satisfaction level in situations in which innovations are occurring that the possibility of the Hawthorne effect be considered. In our research this would imply that the high satisfaction found among primary nurses might be related more to the fact that experimentation occurred—something new and different—and less to the nature of the change (primary nursing). Although data were collected over long-term study of the units, the possibility of high satisfaction resulting from the Hawthorne effect cannot yet be ruled out. Our attitude is basically that one can in fact count on this effect to create a climate of satisfaction, and that satisfaction, by whatever means it is derived, is a positive outcome.

Table 8-1. Nurses' satisfaction with the way their work is organized on primary nursing and other nursing units

Level of satisfaction	Primary nursing units (N = 45)	Case method units (N = 25)	Team nursing units (N = 24)	Functional nursing units (N = 16)
Extremely satisfied	30%	10%	12%	10%
Very satisfied	60%	60%	40%	33%
Moderately satisfied	10%	30%	48%	50%
Slightly satisfied	0	0	0	7%
Not at all satisfied	0	0	0	0

Increased professionalization. A strong prediction about primary nursing units was that it would realize nurses' desires to be patient-centered and quality care–centered. An unexpected but encouraging finding was that primary nursing would increase greatly the professional orientation of nurses. Nurses were questioned about the following:

1. If they considered emotional aspects of patient care to be important
2. If they were more often atuned to *just* getting their work done on time and getting out of the hospital
3. If they considered the patient's needs and desires when hospital policy or physician's orders seemed inappropriate
4. If they often considered what the patient thought and treated him as a unique human being
5. If they were proud of their profession and active in increasing their knowledge of nursing
6. If they saw the importance of acknowledging expertise as opposed to efficient service
7. If they were passive to authority figures who dictated to them what they (the authority figures) considered "good" nursing care

Our bias was that nurses with a high professional orientation as opposed to a bureaucratic orientation would resist bureaucratic standards for efficiency. High professionalism included the following: (1) an orientation toward quality care rather than getting work done quickly; (2) a value on individual patient-centered care versus object-oriented care; and (3) the acknowledgment of expertise, not just length of service.

Primary nurses, more than other nurses, were found to express idealistic rather than programmatic views, to emphasize the emotional side of patient care to a greater degree, and to place more emphasis on quality of performance than on fulfilling job requirements such as being at work on time (Table 8-2).

New graduate nurses on primary nursing units not only maintained their high level of commitment to professional ideals, but their professional outlook also

Table 8-2. Professional orientation of primary nurses and nurses on other units

	Percentage of nurses agreeing or strongly agreeing			
Nurses' attitude	Primary nursing units (N = 45)	Case method units (N = 25)	Team nursing units (N = 24)	Functional nursing units (N = 16)
1 Ideals rather than rules and procedures should be followed	58%	35%	27%	27%
2 Emotional side of patient should be more important than knowing technical skills	31%	19%	12%	0
3 Being at work on time rather than quality care should determine promotion	9%	12%	50%	54%

increased over time. They agreed that a nurse should put her high ideals of quality nursing care into practice, even if hospital rules prohibit it. Their opinion that a knowledge of emotional and social factors in the care of the patient should be more important than a knowledge of specific technical skills (such as how to give an enema) was strengthened. In addition, they agreed that if nurses perform exceptionally well in giving nursing care to patients, they should be considered for promotion, even though they are frequently late for work (Table 8-3).

Responses from new graduates on primary nursing units were favorable compared to graduates employed on other units of the hospitals because not only did other graduates lose certain professional ideologies, but they also were lowest in the ideologies that were being strengthened most in new graduates practicing primary nursing. That is, new graduates on other units deviated from their initial high professional orientation more than new graduates on the primary nursing units. For example, after eight months of employment, they agreed more often than primary nurses that promotion should be largely a factor of the length of experience on the job. Considering all questions asked, they measured lowest in professionalism on those questions that new primary nurses rated highest. Essentially they did not believe that nurses should put their standards and ideals of good nursing care into practice if these in any way conflicted with hospital policies. They did not agree that a knowledge of emotional and social factors in the care of the patient should be more important than a knowledge of specific skills. Also they did not think that nurses, even though they performed exceptionally well as nurses, should be considered for promotion if they were frequently late for work.

Changes in colleague relationships. Leininger[2] aptly stated that as primary nurses become more accountable and responsible for total patient care, some changes in the role sets, functions, and activites of the nurse should be expected, which will affect the roles of other disciplines. In our study not only was there a

Table 8-3. Professional orientation of new graduates on primary nursing and other nursing units

| | Percentage of nurses agreeing or strongly agreeing | | | |
| | Graduates on primary nursing units (N = 15) | | Graduates on team and functional nursing units (N = 13) | |
Nurses' attitudes	Before (1 to 3 months' work experience)	After (8 to 10 months' work experience)	Before (1 to 3 months' work experience)	After (8 to 10 months' work experience)
1 Ideals rather than rules and procedures should be followed	60%	75%	40%	20%
2 Emotional side of patient should be more important than knowing technical skills	1%	50%	0	0
3 Being at work on time rather than quality care should determine promotion	42%	30%	60%	50%

change in the role sets that nurses had about other disciplines, but there was also a definite change in the perceptions of nurses about each other.

Within the primary nursing units in our study that employed L.V.N.s as primary nurses, the status bias previously attached to L.V.N.s and senior staff members was relaxed appreciably. Nurses were "nurses" and were evaluated on the basis of how well they could deliver total patient care. Seniority was important only if it made the staff member a better nurse practitioner. The kind of nurse mattered only from the standpoint of what the staff member was legally licensed to do. Great changes occurred when there were no team leaders, and every nurse, whether an R.N. or L.V.N., acted as a primary nurse for patients.

One outcome that was obvious to everyone was the greater reliance and interaction between staff members as peers. The only staff member elevated to a hierarchical position in the minds of staff nurses was the head nurse or nurse manager. It was important for the head nurse to be knowledgeable about all patient care and to know and coordinate activities of primary nurses on all shifts.

With the exception of the head nurse, other nurses were equal and should be treated as such.

The greatest changes in staff colleague relationships seemed to occur between R.N.s and L.V.N.s who chose to take primary nursing assignments. R.N.s became aware that some L.V.N.s could write better nursing care plans than themselves and could establish effective relationships with patients and patients' families.

According to one L.V.N., there were two major changes in the social interaction of the unit and the degree that her talents were used:

> I feel that with primary nursing I get more credit for what I can do; with team nursing, I was always running errands for other nurses. Now I feel that I have the responsibility for my patient. And he knows this too. That's very important to him. . . . Also with team nursing I always got treated unfairly at break time; sometimes I'd get left all alone on the floor. No R.N.s would be there because they'd take their breaks together. Now I plan my own break to suit my patients. I don't have to wait for the R.N.s to take their break first. . . . I guess I'm more my own boss now.

COMPARISON OF NURSES' PERCEPTIONS BEFORE AND AFTER IMPLEMENTATION OF PRIMARY NURSING

As indicated earlier, there were several strategies in the study of nurses in a primary nursing system, and two strategies have been described already: (1) to compare primary nurses with nurses working under other care modalities and (2) to compare new graduate primary nurses with new graduate team and functional nurses over time. A third strategy is the comparison of nurses' perceptions and attitudes on a nursing unit before and after the implementation of primary nursing care. With this comparison, it is possible to control for any peculiarities of nurses on the unit or the unit itself that would make a difference in the results.

As with the study of patients, this kind of comparison could give more assurance about the expectations of the effects of implementing primary nursing. The findings substantiated those results mentioned thus far.

Nurses on the units before and after the implementation of primary nursing differed in their level of satisfaction. Table 8-4 demonstrates that the level of satisfaction of nurses after the implementation of primary nursing increased significantly. This evidence is supported by many reports from other hospitals revealing that their nurses were very satisfied with primary nursing and did not want to return to team nursing, the case method, or functional nursing.

After the implementation of primary nursing, nurses' professional orientation also changed. Nurses agreed more frequently and strongly with the following professional criteria statements:

1. The nurse should put her ideals of nursing practice into operation, despite rules or procedures that counter these ideals.
2. Giving patients emotional support, which involves addressing oneself to various facets of a patient's well-being, is more important than knowing isolated nursing skills.

They were also more likely to disagree or disagree strongly with the statement

Table 8-4. Nurses' satisfaction with the way their work is organized before and after the implementation of primary nursing

Level of satisfaction	Before primary nursing (N = 45)	After primary nursing (N = 45)
Extremely satisfied	0	10%
Very satisfied	25%	54%
Moderately satisfied	50%	36%
Slightly satisfied	15%	0
Not at all satisfied	10%	0

Table 8-5. Professional orientation of nurses before and after implementation of primary nursing

	Frequency nurses agreed (%)	
Nurses' attitudes	Before primary nursing (N = 45)	After primary nursing (N = 45)
1 Ideals rather than rules and procedures should be followed	20%	50%
2 Emotional side of patient care should be more important than knowing technical skills	15%	50%
3 Being at work on time rather than quality care should influence promotion	50%	15%

that not being at work on time (efficiency) should be a determinant in refusing someone promotion if that person was giving quality care to patients.

SUMMARY AND IMPLICATIONS

In summary, primary nursing is an extremely satisfying nursing care modality from nurses' points of view. An outstanding feature of this kind of nursing care was the opportunity for consistent, in-depth relationships with patients and their families. The chances to be accountable for their patients and to be knowledgeable about a few patients rather than knowing a little about many patients were also reported to be desirable features of primary nursing. It seems obvious that primary nursing should help professional nurses use their skills and broad educational background more freely, should give nurses more feedback about their accomplishments with each patient, and should afford nurses a greater sense of autonomy on the job. For these reasons alone, primary nurses exhibit a higher level of work satisfaction than nurses practicing in other nursing care modalities.

It is equally promising that the primary nursing care system fosters professional values of nurses. Not only are primary nurses more professional in their orientation than team or functional nurses, but they can also increase their professional values even more if they are subjected to the primary system over a period of time. Nurses increased their professional attitudes when they went from team to primary nursing units, and the longer their employment on a primary unit, the greater their professionalism. These findings should be highly inspiring to new graduates who leave their educational programs with an idealistic and professional attitude toward nursing but fall prey to the bureaucratic standards and values of their employing institutions.

Finally, the change in role sets and functions that come with primary nursing have interesting implications for leveling organizational hierarchies in nursing. In cases in which L.V.N.s and R.N.s were given primary nursing assignments, there were opportunities for status confusion. The hierarchical nursing team did not exist, and this fact led many nurses to consider each other on a more equal basis in terms of their skills and knowledge and not in terms of their relative status on the unit.

As anticipated, primary nursing—like any other mode of organized nursing care—has a tremendous impact not only on its clients but also on its participants. Primary nursing constitutes a significant change in nurses' attitudes toward their work, in their actual performance, and in their adherence to certain professional ideologies in nursing.

Perhaps the biggest "pay-off" of primary nursing will be to the baccalaureate program nurse, who has for a long time fought against overwhelming odds. In her account of the new baccalaureate graduate in nursing service, Young suggests why primary nursing may be a welcomed alternative for these nurses:

> The baccalaureate program nurse begins to practice in a hospital bureaucracy in which the way we've always done it shuts the door on any other way. It is a laissez-faire, though easy, substitute for the problem-solving approach on which this nurse was weaned.
>
> There are no nursing care plans. "Report" takes the place of patient conferences. Sitting down to talk to a patient is frowned on. Teaching patients is limited to telling them how to follow the steps of technical procedures—if not already delegated to students or someone employed for that purpose. Discussions with physicians are limited to terse questions and answers about orders. An escort takes the patient to treatment areas. And other health team members are isolated in their own practice areas. The "whole patient" vanishes, and in his place are medicines, treatments, and charts. Patient-centered care disappears into the morass of daily routine. The baccalaureate nurse's most precious commodities—the carefully nurtured skills in interpersonal relationships, problem solving, and application of scientific principles—may be repressed, for they are not negotiable.
>
> Instead, hospital supervisory personnel are confused about the new graduate's questioning attitude. Sometimes, they are irritated by her reluctance to accept the status quo. They consider her inability to manage a large patient assignment immediately a serious liability and compare her unfavorably with the diploma program graduate who does—without questioning. Moreover, they may see nursing primarily in its technical component, and pressed by the responsibility for supervising the care of many patients by an insufficient number of nurses, they deplore the young baccalaureate nurse's initial lack of technical proficiency.

In time, the baccalaureate nurse who persists in her desire to work with patients takes one of two routes. Geared to learning rapidly, she quickly becomes skilled in the hospital's routines, perhaps a little resentful that she has been put at a disadvantage. Another nurse, no different. Or, she seeks a position in some other field, often public health, in which she as the freedom to make judgments, solve problems, and seek solutions. The feeling of deprivation which she experienced in the hospital bureaucracy has driven her away from the hospital. The satisfactions of patient care she had realized as a student have become a delusion.*

---

*From Young, L. S.: The new baccalaureate graduate in nursing service, Nursing Outlook **14:**50, Nov., 1966.

REFERENCES

1. Leininger, M. M., Little, D. E., and Carnevali, D.: Primex, American Journal of Nursing **72:**1274-1277, 1972.
2. Leininger, M. M.: The culture concept and its relevance to nursing. In Auld, M. E., and Birum, L. H., editors: The challenge of nursing: a book of readings, St. Louis, 1973, The C. V. Mosby Co., pp. 39-46.

SUGGESTED READINGS

Berkowitz, N. H., and Malone, M.: Intra-professional conflict, Nursing Forum **3:**65-69, Winter, 1968.

Blau, P. M.: Bureaucracy in modern society, New York, 1956, Random House.

Corwin, R. C., and Taves, M. J.: Some concomitants of bureaucratic and professional conceptions of the nurse role, Nursing Research **11:**227, Fall, 1962.

Fielding, V.: New team plan frees nurses to nurse, Modern Hospital **5:**122-124, May, 1969.

Graves, H. H.: Can nursing shed bureaucracy? American Journal of Nursing **71:**491-495, 1971.

Harrington, H., and Theis, C.: Institutional factors perceived by baccalaureate graduates as influencing their performance as staff nurses, Nursing Research **17:**228-235, May-June, 1968.

Hayter, J.: A follow-up study of graduates of the baccalaureate degree program in nursing, Nursing Research **12:**45-47, Winter, 1963.

Kramer, M.: New graduate speaks, American Journal of Nursing **66:**2420-2424, 1966.

Kramer, M.: The new graduate speaks again, American Journal of Nursing **69:**1903-1907, 1969.

Meyer, G. R.: Tenderness and technique: nursing values in transition. Industrial Relations Monograph No. 6, Los Angeles, 1960, Institute of Human Relations, University of California Press.

Scott, W. R.: Professionals in bureaucracies. In Volmer, H., and Mills, D., editors: Professionalization, Englewood Cliffs, N. J., 1966, Prentice-Hall, Inc., pp. 265-274.

chapter 9

EFFECTS OF PRIMARY NURSING ON RELATED PERSONNEL AND SYSTEMS

One could hardly expect that a major change in the organization of nursing care would not affect related personnel and systems within the institution. As the role set, functions, and activities, as well as the accountability of the nurse change, so do the roles of related disciplines and systems. Thus change in a nursing care modality would seem to have implications for other systems changing. Top administrators, physicians, and personnel from various auxiliary services, who also serve the patient either directly or indirectly, may feel the impact of primary nursing care.

For these reasons a study of the effects of primary nursing on attitudes and perceptions of other systems and personnel in the hospital was undertaken. Although it was not possible to survey every service that would logically feel the impact of primary nursing, two key groups were considered: administrators and physicians. A secondary focus of this study was to assess the feasibility or cost-effectiveness of primary nursing care, since this issue would seem to affect the physician's and administrator's support for this change in nursing care.

THE STUDY

To survey attitudes of physicians and administrators about primary nursing, we utilized several modes of data collection. Surveys to selected hospitals known to be practicing primary nursing were sent to an administrator of the hospital, usually the director of nurses. This survey tapped attitudes toward primary nursing, as well as inquired about the cost-effectiveness of primary nursing compared to other nursing care modalities used by that hospital. In addition, several informal interviews were held with selected administrators in institutions that seemed to be well on the way to implementing primary nursing successfully.

These informal interviews also provided some statistical data from the various nursing service offices regarding the cost of units in nursing salaries, the number of sick days and absences, and the amount of overtime without pay of primary nurses as opposed to nurses working under the case method, functional, or team nursing systems.

A formal questionnaire was designed to ascertain physicians' opinions and attitudes about primary nursing care units. This questionnaire was sent to physicians who had patients on primary nursing units and physicians who had patients on team, functional, and case method nursing units.

Physicians were asked to comment about how satisfied they were with the nursing care and to list advantages and disadvantages of the nursing modality. Approximately 60 percent of the questionnaires were returned, representing a good distribution between the different kinds of units. The questionnaires were administered in the initial stages of implementing primary nursing, and therefore responses indicate physicians' attitudes during one time period only.

Physicians' responses from the hospitals resulted in a total sample of fifty physicians with patients on functional nursing, case method nursing, team nursing, and primary nursing units. Informal comments of physicians to staff nurses were recorded to supplement physician's responses to the formal questionnaire.

PREDICTIONS ABOUT EFFECTS OF PRIMARY NURSING ON RELATED PERSONNEL AND SYSTEMS

A major assumption of this study was that primary nursing would be regarded with mixed emotions by related hospital and medical personnel. First, implementation of primary nursing required these personnel to change, and change is difficult. In addition, it required change in personnel who did not initiate the change and who would never know the tremendous satisfaction that primary nurses would feel with the change. Physicians and others, then, would not reap the benefits that nurses would. Because of these points, it was expected that primary nursing, at least in the beginning and periodically throughout its development, would be received with mixed emotions. These mixed emotions would persist despite attempts of unit-level nursing staff to co-opt related personnel in the change process. Co-optation would serve only to superficially involve others and would require a great deal of energy to maintain. The chances of co-optation being neglected as a strategy and of doubt arising in both administrators' and physicians' minds were great. Therefore the attitudes of physicians and administrators should fluctuate and indicate a degree of ambivalence throughout the change process.

It should be recalled that the outcomes of primary nursing are many, including the following:
1. Increased accountability of the nurse for total patient care
2. A more rational basis for delivery of nursing care (that is, the nurse who knows the most about the patient is responsible for his care)
3. Individualized and personalized patient care
4. Increased equality among nursing staff

Although these outcomes have some redeeming features in the eyes of physicians and administrators, they pose some problems as well. Depending on the individual physician, these features can cause a great deal of alarm. The problems in part are related to the complimentary role relationships of physicians and registered nurses that have existed up to this time.

As noted, under the primary nursing system the relationship between nurse and patient become a great deal more personal and cohesive because of the increase in nursing accountability and continuity and the nurse's attempt to individualize patient care. As the relationship between the nurse and patient becomes more cohesive and instrumental to the well-being of the patient, the relationship between physician and patient may become secondary to the patient and arouse some professional jealousy in the physician.

Some physicians believe that they *should be* and *are* the primary guardians of their patients while they are in the hospital. A physician may execute his guardian responsibilities by intervening between the patient and the nurse or, for that matter, between the patient and the dietary service or between the hospital billing system and the patient. In this way, the physician takes on the role of "host" in an institution in which he has much authority but only sporadically visits. He may actually view himself as the key representative for the patient while the patient is in *his* hospital.

Although a variety of health care personnel, as well as the patient's family, may act as the patient's guardians, nurses and physicians probably are the chief occupants of such a role. Since primary nursing sets up a close relationship between the patient and nurse, the physician is less likely to act as the patient's chief guardian. The nurse's usurping of the physician's role causes him to change his perception of his role and may cause him to come in conflict with the primary nurse. Primary nursing then may be perceived as a threat to physicians.

Physicians may view primary nursing as a threat for other reasons. Since they know a great deal about their patients, primary nurses may have knowledge that physicians do not have. Because of this added knowledge, nurses may be better able to make good judgments about patient care. A physician who prides himself on knowing more than nurses about patients may find the growing expertise of the nurse a threat to his status and self-concept as a physician.

Finally, the fact that the status of R.N.s and L.V.N.s is more equalized under a primary nursing system may be threatening to physicians. Some physicians prefer to deal only with registered nurses. For various reasons physicians have helped establish and cooperated in the hierarchy in nursing by regarding L.V.N.s as "not *real* nurses." Primary nursing does not arbitrarily set up a hierarchical division between L.V.N.s and R.N.s, and, as a result, physicians may be dismayed, confused, and disenchanted. The physician who wants to confer with his patient's nurse will have to work closely with the primary nurse, and the primary nurse just may be an L.V.N. and not an R.N.

The physician's attitude of hesitancy may be shared by administrators. Depending on the philosophy of the nursing office, the courage of the director of nurses, and the strength of the physician group, administrators may feel equally uncomfortable.

Generally, administrators are extremely concerned about physicians' opinions of nursing care. Administrators must keep their physicians happy so that the hospital will receive their patients, thus maintaining an adequate hospital census. They must hear and mediate physicians' complaints, as well as plan new and innovative approaches to nursing. Thus if the physician is unhappy, the administration may be unhappy.

Other consequences of primary nursing besides physicians' reactions may cause administrators further dismay. Although increased accountability of the nurse, can result in increased effectiveness and efficiency of the nurse as well as increased nurse satisfaction, it has one disquieting consequence. It usually makes the "bad" nurse appear "bad." Finding good nurses who will be good primary nurses is a problem. Therefore, if primary nurses have not been chosen wisely, administrators may face more complaints about individual nurses.

Also, increased accountability and professionalism for nurses can cause them to question and challenge hospital policies. If administrators are not ready for self-assertive staff nurses, they may be threatened by a change in staff reactions to standardized policies and procedures.

Finally, increased equality among different levels of nurses can result in financial as well as legal problems. L.V.N.s in a primary nursing system may not accept a differentiation in wages, especially since the differences in responsibilities of R.N.s and L.V.N.s are more vague than with a team nursing system. If they are "primary nurses like R.N.s," why are their wages different? Not only do administrators have to supervise the increased accountability of L.V.N.s from a legal point of view, but they also need to have ready answers for the different financial treatment of L.V.N.s under a primary nursing system. For these reasons, administrators as well as physicians should feel some resentment toward a change, particularly toward a change to primary nursing.

Features of primary nursing that should be offsetting negative reactions of administrators and physicians may cause these groups to be happy with the system.

The fact that primary nursing provides a more rational basis for delivery of nursing care can be welcomed by physicians and administrators alike. Rational delivery means that there is a nurse who is knowledgeable about an individual patient, and she or he is also the person delivering the care. Nursing care will be more successful, and physicians will have knowledgeable nurses attending their patients.

According to physicians' comments recorded by Manthey and Kramer,[1] physicians believe that primary nurses have a much better knowledge of patients and the subtle changes that occur, and this is important to them. This is primarily because primary nurses have seen patients over a period of days and have a basis for comparison from one day to the next.

If nursing care is more successful, errors may decrease. More knowledgeable nurses may be a great relief to the physician who has too many patients and too little time to know his patients. Physicians may come to depend on the nurse to a greater degree to help in making professional judgments. In addition, with the increase in accountability of the nurse, physicians need not be subjected to the perennial "passing the buck" system among nursing staff. They can rest assured that the person who gets the order will carry it out and will also be the person responsible for the outcome.

Increased continuity and coordination of patient care are also advantages for physicians. If a physician gives an order, he can rest assured that the same nurse will carry it out and be responsible. In addition, the same nurse may give him an evaluation of what happened and plan future interventions with him.

Personalized and individualized nursing care also has positive outcomes for the physician and administrator. Personalized and individualized care is more likely to make the patient happy. A happy patient makes for a satisfied physician and a satisfied administration, provided the care given is adequate and safe. A consistent humanistic and individualized approach by the nurse, then, can be viewed by both administrators and physician as desirable.

In summary, for many reasons both administrative and physician groups experience repercussions when changes occur in nursing care modalities. As pointed out, the outcomes of primary nursing can cause both negative and positive reactions in physicians and administrators; thus these groups should experience a great deal of ambivalence about primary nursing. Their feelings may fluctuate from positive to negative or may be positive and negative at the same time.

ATTITUDES OF PHYSICIANS ABOUT PRIMARY NURSING

A review of fifty physicians' opinions about the different nursing care modalities (functional, case, team, and primary nursing) produced some interesting results. As expected, opinions of the physicians were mixed, and individual physicians varied their remarks about how satisfied they were and what they thought the advantages to be.

A general satisfaction measure for all physicians indicated that physicians were not especially more satisfied with primary nursing as compared to the team, functional, or case methods. Table 9-1 indicates that whereas 90 percent of physicians evaluating the functional and case methods were very or extremely satisfied with the nursing care, 85 percent of physicians evaluating primary nursing and 80 percent evaluating team nursing were very or ex-

Table 9-1. Satisfaction of physicians with nursing care

Level of satisfaction	Primary nursing (N = 15)	Case method (N = 8)	Functional method (N = 7)	Team nursing (N = 20)
Extremely satisfied	15%	20%	20%	6.7%
Very satisfied	70%	70%	70%	73.3%
Moderately satisfied	15%	10%	10%	20%
Slightly satisfied	0	0	0	0
Not at all satisfied	0	0	0	0

tremely satisfied. Although primary nursing tended to make more physicians extremely satisfied than team nursing, the functional and case methods were extremely satisfying to more physicians than was primary or team nursing care.

The responses on this global measure of satisfaction indicate that the skill of the individual nurse may be of chief importance to the physician as opposed to the system of care. In this study the functional and case method units surveyed were specialty and intensive care units. These units had been staffed by nurses who were handpicked for the unit. This factor contaminates the study results, since, obviously, "better skilled" nurses may have been placed on these units, and the technical skills of nurses are extremely important to physicians. As one physician explained: "We physicians make distinctions only between bad and good nurses. . . . Most of us don't express a direct interest in how nursing care is dispensed unless something goes wrong. . . ."[1]

These global evaluations of physicians do not necessarily fit their specific responses to open-ended questions on the same questionnaire and in informal interviews that physicians held with the nursing staff on primary nursing units. Although their answers to the satisfaction question reveal that these physicians were not appreciably more satisfied with primary nursing compared to other modes of nursing care, further comments revealed that it was not actually primary nursing causing them to be hesitant.

Physicians were asked to point out advantages and disadvantages of primary nursing and those commenting about primary nursing units did not identify disadvantages that could be directly associated with primary nursing per se. Any negative comments that were made referred to the following categories of complaints:

1. Personal characteristics of individual nurses (such as appearance, mannerisms, age, race)
2. Staff familiarity with nonroutine orders
3. Staff understanding of the disease process
4. Understaffing
5. Promptness in recording orders

These comments could be addressed to any nursing staff, regardless of the mode of nursing care practiced on a unit. For this reason these comments have limited value in assessing physicians' impressions of a change in nursing modality.

The content of physicians' comments on advantages of primary nursing was much more revealing. Physicians' positive regard for primary nursing also grew over time and as they became more familiar with the new modality. The most frequently named advantages were as follows:

1. Stability of nursing care, with the same nurse caring for the physician's patient day in and day out
2. The nurse's knowledge of the physician's plans for treatment
3. Personalized concern and attention to the patient's needs, as well as intellectual interest in patients

4. Good communication from shift to shift and good communication with the physician
5. Generally good climate to work in because of the motivated staff and other factors

(The two most frequently mentioned advantages in this list were Nos. 3 and 4.)

The only overt signs of ambivalence and competition that could be attributed to the change in the nursing care modality were physicians' increased sense of curiosity and their displayed sense of humor. Several physicians became increasingly interested in learning what primary nurses did as opposed to other nurses. A few decided to become involved in the teaching of primary nurses. One physician commented jokingly: "The only thing wrong with primary nursing is that a physician is not in charge! Heh, heh."

It is interesting to note that in the face of change and competition with nurses, physicians will repeatedly manifest the traditional attitudes of subservient relationships, as demonstrated in the statement "things will be okay if *we* can just control what nurses do" and the offer "let *me* teach you."

ATTITUDES OF ADMINISTRATORS
ABOUT PRIMARY NURSING

Administrators from seven of nine hospitals implementing primary nursing responded to a general survey about how they were implementing this change and what their attitudes were about it. In each case, administrators endorsed primary nursing as a valid and workable way of organizing nursing care. Whereas nursing directors and assistant administrators emphasized the cost-effectiveness issue and assignment and organization of staff, in-service coordinators and supervisors commented idealistically about outcomes for nurses and patients and the relationship between nurses and patients.

Administrators described various features about primary nursing that they thought needed special attention. Two consistent criteria for a workable system were (1) a healthy ratio of R.N.s to other nursing personnel and (2) the opportunity to handpick the nurses who would be primary nurses. These concerns were interpreted as reflecting the consequence that under primary nursing, nurses are more accountable and are in positions to make independent decisions. Thus "good" nurses should be placed in primary nursing positions, since "bad" nurses appear worse in primary nursing situations.

Although there was more equality between L.V.N.s and R.N.s, this was not mentioned as a problem. This may be due to the fact that the majority of units were using high ratios of R.N.s to L.V.N.s and that the L.V.N.s on the primary nursing units were also handpicked.

Increased nurse self-esteem and status conflict with physicians were not mentioned by administrators in the formal questionnaires. These problems did, however, become evident over long-term observation and interviews with administrators in two hospitals. The main concerns of administrators were that primary nurses may come across as "super-nurses" to physicians and that this would be threatening to physicians. At the same time, administrators, especially nursing administrators, were ambivalent. On the one hand, they were coaching primary nurses not to offend or threaten doctors; on the other hand, they were saying: "Show doctors what *we* can do." Their ambivalence about primary nurses was probably conveyed in some way to both nursing staff and physician groups.

Data about the cost-effectiveness of primary nursing were gathered from various statistics comparing the operation of primary care units with other case method, functional, and team nursing units in the hospitals. These data had been collected as a natural administrative process of the hospitals. As indicated earlier, it was thought that the cost-effectiveness of primary nursing as compared to other nursing modalities would affect the attitudes of both physicians and administrators.

The statistics from the nursing offices represented various aspects of the administrative effectiveness of primary nursing, including (1) the cost in terms of salaries to nurses on primary nursing care units as compared to the cost on other units and (2) the number of sick days and number of absences of nurses on primary nursing units as compared to other units. These statistics were compiled over a period of one and one-half years. Any discrepancies resulting from periodic lapses in hospital census taking or seasonal variations in attendance were controlled by this longitudinal study. Also, each unit compared was compared with another unit during the same time period, thereby making the comparison a fair and valid one.

It was important to know just what primary nursing units, with highly individualized care and extremely satisfied nursing staff working in an atmosphere breeding greater professionalism, was costing compared to other units and how administrators would view the cost-effectiveness issue.

Without too much reflection, it was assumed that units employing greater numbers of registered nurses practicing primary nursing (in which one nurse had five patients at the most) would be extremely costly. Also, a unit manned solely by registered nurses, as was one initial experimental unit with young graduates, would definitely put the hospital "in the red." Obviously, whatever is ideal is more expensive or, at least, should be. This logic summarizes the belief of administrators at the outset of implementing primary nursing. Administrators' attitudes toward primary nursing would be influenced by this logic, which may account for the initial caution and hesitancy of administrators to experiment with primary nursing on more than a limited basis.

However, in a comparative analysis of an initial experimental unit and other units, it was found that the same total number of R.N.s, L.V.N.s, and aides could be employed on another unit of comparable size as new graduate R.N.s on an experimental unit.

Essentially, this was because the new graduate R.N.s were first-level staff nurses on the pay scale. Many L.V.N.s on the other units were getting as much if not more money than the new graduate R.N.s. None of the hospitals surveyed reported an increase in the cost of operating primary nursing care units compared to team, functional, or case method units, and three reported that it was less costly. Administrators from one hospital explained that they were spending less money because they were using 10,000 nursing hours per year less with primary nursing. According to administrators from another hospital, they were saving on nursing hours per patient day. Although their primary nursing units had a higher proportion of R.N.s whose salaries were higher than other nursing personnel (as measured by hours per patient day), the units were operating much more effectively and with less cost than other units (as measured by cost per patient day).

Some administrators reported greater productivity on primary nursing care units as compared to other units in the hospital. The high morale of nurses on these units indicated that for them, overtime was not a burden to be avoided but was accepted and was even considered necessary when the time could be spent on writing primary nursing care plans, making home visits, or working on special projects. Not only did the high morale of nurses lead to more overtime service without financial reimbursement, but it also provided greater continuity of service. Nurses on one experimental unit had approximately one half the number of sick hours and absences as nurses on the other units.

According to administrators' views of the cost-effectiveness issue, primary nursing would be desirable to them.

SUMMARY

Although administrators' and physicians' opinions about primary nursing were not overwhelmingly and enthusiastically supportive of this change, certain conclusions can be drawn with some degree of confidence.

It is highly likely that physicians and administrators would endorse primary nursing more often than not and endorse it over most other modes of dispensing nursing care delivery.

Primary nursing offers the features of personalized nursing care, a more rational basis for delivery of nursing care, and increased accountability of the nurse, which are all highly desirable to physician and administrator groups. These features promise happy patients and good communication between a knowledgeable nurse and the doctor. Since primary nursing apparently does not cost more than other modes of nursing care, in the opinion of administrators, it has a good chance of survival.

When a mode of nursing care produces more satisfaction in nurses and greater individualized patient care, in addition to satisfying efficiency and effectiveness criteria, it can no longer be ignored or put aside as a "passing fancy." This means that physicians and administrators will consider seriously whether they want or will endorse primary nursing as a change.

In this chapter several reactions were identified that may cause both administrators and physicians to be ambivalent toward this change. Although physicians and administrators did not appear to have overwhelming negative or positive feelings toward primary nursing, there were good indications of substantial support. The extent that administrators and physicians are clearly ambivalent and the basis of their ambivalence are interesting and worth mentioning. At this point, most of the consequences of primary nursing are likely to arouse reactions in physicians and administrators. Perhaps the most controversial consequences are (1) the increased accountability and autonomy of nurses and (2) the leveling among nursing staff.

Administrators and physicians are only a small, although admittedly important part of the work system analysis. Further studies of reactions of other personnel and systems in the hospital (and outside the hospital) to the primary nursing care modality are important and need to be undertaken.

REFERENCE

1. Manthey, M., and Kramer, M.: A dialogue on primary nursing, Nursing Forum **9:**356-379, 1970.

SUGGESTED READINGS

Etzioni, A.: Modern organizations, Englewood Cliffs, N. J., 1964, Prentice-Hall, Inc.

Etzioni, A., editor: The semi-professions and their organization, New York, 1969, The Free Press.

Freidson, E.: Profession of medicine, New York, 1971, Dodd, Mead & Co.

Goode, William J.: Community within a community: the professions, American Sociological Review **22:**195-200, 1957.

Scott, W. R., and Dornbruch, S.: Evaluation and authority, New York, 1973, McGraw-Hill Book Co.

Thompson, James: Hierarchy, specialization, and organizational conflict, Administrative Science Quarterly **5:**521-526, 1961.

Thompson, James: Organizations in action, New York, 1967, McGraw-Hill Book Co.

chapter 10

SUMMARY AND DISCUSSIONS
OF PRIMARY NURSING

One of the most valuable outcomes of consulting in the area of primary nursing has been the relevancy and the quality of questions asked. These questions deal with what we attempted to implement and study at various hospitals, in addition to what primary nursing means and what its limitations are. These questions reflect more generally the nursing profession's acceptance of primary nursing and primary care and its struggle to give this care modality a meaningful context in the education of nurses.

The intention of this chapter is to present some of the more provocative questions, as well as the answers and discussion, stimulated by conversations with administrators, physicians, nurses, and nurse educators. This chapter will identify and highlight some of the most provocative questions asked.

Are you against team nursing?

Because we can never be totally for or against anything out of context, this question always makes us a little uncomfortable.

First, there is more than one kind of team nursing. As a matter of fact, some team nursing methods resemble primary nursing in that some nurses on the team may have total responsibility for patient care to a few individual patients. So, let us clarify our position.

There are several criteria for a good nursing care modality. One criterion is to unify or make holistic the patient's care to minimize the fragmentation of his care. The second criterion is placement of nursing care at the patient's side to avoid the pyramiding of nursing care delivery and nurses' preoccupation with nursing hierarchy.

The fragmentation of care that generally occurs with team nursing tends to prevent total patient care by one nurse. Also team leading generally introduces a value on nursing hierarchy by superimposing vertical positions of authority. Except in rare cases, nurses not only worry about how good their care is to patients (including patients they give only partial care to sometimes) but also whether their team likes them and what the team leader will tell the head nurse about their performance.

As opposed to any other modality, primary nursing would most likely be chosen as meeting the criteria of holism and patient-oriented delivery. Team nursing and functional nursing, both of which tend to fragment care and superimpose a hierarchy in delivering that care, leave something to be desired.

If you're against teaming in nursing, are you against teaming in general?

Now this is a tricky question. Usually what is meant by "teaming in general" is professional health teams; thus the second question is actually "Are you against professional health teams?"

It is apparent that the first and second questions are different, at least in some respects. The purpose of teaming, as we conceive it and in its most idealized form, is to consolidate professional talents in behalf of the patient. Theoretically the patient should benefit not only from the fact that "two (professional) heads are better than one" but also from the fact that each professional brings to the patient unique skills and talents, which, if combined, would provide him optimal health care services.

Our attitudes about the drawbacks of the hierarchical relationships and fragmentation of patient care associated with teaming do not change. On the other hand, a paraprofessional team is both appropriate and necessary. Basically, we see great benefits of professional relationships in behalf of quality patient care, involving the nurse, physician, clergy, family, social worker, occupational therapist, physical therapist, dietician and psychologist.

Primary nursing incorporates the health team concept in its implementation (see Chapter 4). Primary nursing provides the health team with a nurse who is knowledgeable about the patient, who has established a one-to-one relationship with him (sometimes prior to his admission to the hospital), and who is an excellent resource for feedback to the professional team. The primary nurse is also an excellent agent to induce change in the patient that is in keeping with the goals of the total health team.

Is primary nursing the same as primary care?

This question and a number of others focus on the specific operational features and aim at a clearer definition of primary nursing. Basically primary nursing and primary care are different concepts. However, they are frequently confused, even in the most sophisticated nursing circles.

Primary care means that the initial assessment, diagnosis, and treatment (depending on the nature of the treatment) is done by a nurse who has the necessary skills and training to work in the practitioner capacity. Primary nursing, although it may include primary care, is more global and comprehensive. Primary nurses may do the primary care of their patients, but they are not limited to primary care. They function to give holistic patient care and may participate in the follow-up of patients beyond the initial assessment stage.

As discussed earlier, primary nursing can best be distinguished if it is compared with functional or team nursing. One nurse is responsible for the total care of an individual patient as opposed to a team of nurses having this responsibility.

Table 10-1. Comparison of primary care with primary nursing

	Primary care	*Primary nursing care*
Practitioner	May be physician, nurse, or other health professional delegated and/or licensed to provide initial diagnosis and treatment of patient	Always a nurse
Setting	Clinics, hospitals, private practice	Clinics, hospitals, public health departments
Focus	Health and illness oriented; may be highly specific to patient's problem and may or may not include family and holistic view of patient; can be short-term, crisis-oriented care by an initial practitioner, with follow-up by a second practitioner	Patient (person) oriented; always includes both patient and family as well as factors affecting the patient, including socioemotional, cultural, and economic; care is sometimes short term, but follow-up is usually by the same nurse who makes the initial contact with the patient
Goals or objectives	In health profession: 1. Initial assessment and treatment of the patient who usually has acute illness 2. Better coverage of health problems by persons capable of making initial assessment and and treatment of patients	In nursing: 1. Continuity of patient care 2. Comprehensive patient care 3. Patient-centered care 4. Accountability for patient care 5. Coordinated nursing care

One can easily confuse primary care and primary nursing, and it is not always important to make the distinction. But it is important to keep in mind the more comprehensive and "long-term" features of primary nursing, which are different from primary care per se, whether we are talking about the hospital setting or nursing in the community at large. (See Table 10-1 for a comparison of primary care and primary nursing.)

Is primary nursing merely getting the nurse back to the bedside—for total care of the patient?

This question usually tests our sensitivity. Although if given a chance the interrogator would probably reword his question, we cannot help responding immediately, "How can any nursing be *merely* getting the nurse back to the bedside?"

Here, the old questions of "What is nursing?" and "What should nursing be?" as well as question of the values attached to nursing at the bedside, raise their persistent heads.

Our opinion is that nursing is and should remain a function of meeting the needs of patients for total nursing care as nurses perceive them through *direct* interaction with their patients. The adequacy of a nurse's assessment, interventions, and evaluation of nursing care depend on transactions with the patient and his family. A great many of these transactions occur in the minute-to-minute exchanges between the patient and the nurse, who is "at his side," wherever it may be.

Doesn't primary nursing foster dependency of patients on nurses?

Research does show that with primary nursing care, patients are treated as special, and therefore it is conceivable that they may strive to maintain their relationship with their primary nurses beyond their need for such a special relationship.

More important to acknowledge here, however, is that few clients at the height of their illness or crisis and at the beginning of their hospitalization do not benefit from a close one-to-one relationship with a health professional. Patients are dependent at initial stages of their hospitalization; why not recognize the fact? One patient explained that what was most terrifying was when the nurse did not perceive that the patient was dependent on the nurse.

This one-to-one relationship makes sense in terms of what is known of an individual's initial adjustment to hospitalization and also in terms of his reaction to stress and illness. Dependency in these cases may be justified if not encouraged by nurses. It is usually not until the last stage of hospitalization (when discharge is imminent) or in the tertiary phases of illness that independence is expected and encouraged. Only at these times are patients expected to truly reactivate their desires to be sociable and to speak up for themselves and protect themselves from possible neglect by nursing or medical staff. If the patient is dependent, it should not be pretended that anything other than a dependency relationship with the nurse is appropriate.

In addition, when the client is ready to be more independent, and the nurse perceives the need for him to be more independent, primary nursing will not be a barrier. Primary nurses can gear their interactions with patients to deliberately foster independence if it is appropriate for the patient. They, more than others, will perceive more quickly and be able to respond more consistently to patients' needs either for greater independence or dependence.

How does primary nursing relate to the question of nurses' accountability for patient care?

Currently accountability is a popular topic in nursing. Probably no other known mode of organizing nursing care promises as much nurse accountability as primary nursing. Nurses cannot be totally accountable for the care of individual patients if individual patient care is divided among two or more nurses within a shift and among four or more nurses within a twenty-four–hour period. It has finally been realized in nursing that the patient is composed of interrelated parts and that no one treatment or intervention can be viewed or evaluated in isolation from other treatments and interventions. Why then would nurses who are administering medications be expected to be accountable if they do not have the responsibility of comprehensive patient care? Could nurses who do not see patients other than at hours that they pass medicines truly be accountable for meeting patients' needs for a more appropriate medication regimen? Are nurses who give only a portion of total care to patients actually committed to the overall well-being of patients? We contend that even if nurses wanted to be accountable, it is virtually impossible for them to be. They cannot perceive enough and check their assessments enough to be held accountable for even the "isolated" regimens of patients' medications. Medication regimens cannot be isolated as specific unrelated tasks. But even if they were, it would be impossible for the nurse to be held accountable for evaluating patients' reactions to medicines as a treatment program.

It would seem that if accountability for patient care means accountability for total patient care (and we argue that true accountability is just that), then primary nursing as opposed to team or functional nursing promises more. Not only are primary nurses more committed to the overall well-being of their patients, but they also have the responsibility for total care; this responsibility is not shared with several other nurses.

Isn't primary nursing impractical?

Just what is meant by impractical? Does it mean too inefficient? For whom is it impractical?

Usually this question is asked with nursing administration in mind and has to do with efficiency and cost issues; that is, how cost-effective is primary nursing? As pointed out in Chapter 9, primary nursing is not any less efficient than other modes of nursing care, according to administrators. Primary nursing costs no more than other modes of nursing care. Some hospitals reported that it was less expensive than team nursing, with respect to total number of nursing care hours provided patients. Because primary nursing increases the morale of nursing staff, it may also increase productivity in that more work is done by the same number of nurses. Thus primary nursing is apparently not impractical when considering the cost-effectiveness of a nursing modality.

In fact, if the goal is to achieve high-quality and comprehensive patient care, then primary nursing is the most efficient means because it saves time in affecting adjustment to hospitalization and illness, and fewer nursing hours are spent to come to a full comprehensive assessment of any one patient and his family. Given the high cost of hospital and health care in general, one would anticipate that the public will want more for their money. Hospitals that can compete for patients on the basis of better individualized patient care will come out on top of the high-cost crunch.

What problems would we have if we wanted to implement primary nursing and what does this mean to nursing education and nursing administration?

Because we generally appear biased in our positive esteem for primary nursing, we generally become overconscientious about looking at the disadvantages and constraints of primary nursing. By far, one of the greatest problems of implementing primary nursing is getting qualified nursing staff to operate as head nurses (or nurse managers) and primary nurses with the primary nursing system.

Primary nurses must possess high-level nursing knowledge and skills, which in many instances are not put to use with team nursing. They must have an ability to assess, plan, implement, and evaluate the total care they give to individual patients. Above all, they need to be able to relate to patients and to patients' families in an intense nurse-client relationship. Primary nurses must be committed to giving each patient what, ideally, he deserves and never perceive their work as mundane, repetitious, or dull. They must be willing to accept total responsibility for each of their patients and view this responsibility in the patient's context of health and illness when his care is not confined to any one hospitalization. They must approach the patient "where he is," never superimposing the fact that they are there to give medicines, administer a treatment, or change his bed. In summary, much is expected of primary nurses not only in terms of knowledge and skill but also in terms of commitment to professional nursing.

All nurses are not prepared to meet this challenge. In addition, not all nurses can sustain the pace of primary nursing at its ideal level of implementation.

We experimented initially with new graduates because nursing education seemed to foster the idealism necessary for primary nursing. It is not clear whether the level of graduate is important, but it is likely that baccalaureate nursing programs provide a good environment for producing potential beginning primary nurses. It was also our experience that a select group of new diploma graduates and associate arts (A.A.) graduates, given the proper environment and reinforcement, can also be good primary nurses.

Generally, nursing programs as well as in-service education programs should provide opportunities for students to learn the value of giving comprehensive patient care, of having a professional orientation toward one's career, and of never doing second best for patients. Patient care and not directing one's peers should be regarded as the ultimate reward.

The other necessary components of a good primary nursing curriculum (that is, opportunities to develop a keen ability to assess, plan, intervene, and evaluate a variety of patients' needs) should be viewed on an equal basis with these opportunities. Nursing education traditionally begins with students being intensely involved with a small number of patients and then shifts its emphasis to leadership and management of peers and subordinates—as if that was more important and required greater skill. Why forsake the beginning approach to teaching students if the profession wants to ensure students' retention of values necessary for primary nursing care?

What is the role of the head nurse or nurse manager on a primary nursing unit?

One common misunderstanding is that head nurses sit in their offices at the desk "managing their staff." Although they are managers of staff, head nurses do not have the alibi to be deskbound. On the contrary, one way for head nurses to be aware of the needs of their staff and respond to the minute-to-minute manifestations of these needs is to be available at the desk, down the hall, in the conference room—literally everywhere that their staff may be. Head nurses must be accessible. But they must not confuse their accessibility with a lack of faith in their staffs' ability. If there is anything more defeating to primary nursing, it is head nurses who allow for staff accountability for the patient care and surreptitiously take it away. The basic premise of the head nurse role is undermined by the head nurse who constantly responds by taking over patient care with a "let me show you how," which indicates the attitude "I feel I know better and can do better than you." Head nurses must enable others (staff members) to increase and utilize full accountability; they must not take the accountability away by taking over staff members' assignments.

What then does the head nurse do when a nurse asks for help or when a nurse is believed to be unsafe?

These are basically two separate issues. First, head nurses must problem solve with their staff. They can facilitate staff effectiveness by asking: "What did you see?," "How is that a problem?," and "What are you going to do now?" Second, if a staff nurse is deemed unsafe, the head nurse must restrict that nurse's delivery of patient care by limiting either the number of patients or the kind of patients, depending on the nurse's areas of weakness and strength.

Thus, although head nurses reinforce accountability in their staff members by not "doing it for them," they do not, on the other hand, relinquish their responsibility to monitor and assign nurses according to their growth needs.

Frequently, there is a fine line between reinforcing responsibility of staff for their patients and at the same time accepting the responsibility of managing a unit. Head nurses must achieve a balance whereby they do not, overtly or covertly, take away that which they intend to impart.

What are you suggesting—that A.A. and diploma graduates are the primary nurses of the future (and that the head nurse will have a B.S. degree; the supervisor, an M.S. degree; and the director of nursing, a Ph.D. degree)?

This question is infrequently asked but important. It mirrors the present over-consciousness of the profession with degrees and levels. Even when we try to avoid a discussion of degrees in nursing and the implications of "what degree occupies what position," we inevitably find ourselves at some point debating the issue, since our position is that the degree does not occupy the position. Many factors including personal characteristics, education, and experience, go into making a good primary nurse, head nurse, supervisor, and director in a primary nursing care system.

An important criterion for a good primary nurse, in addition to degrees, experience, job preparation, and personal characteristics, is the personal affinity of the individual for the job. For example, when selecting primary nurses, one must consider whether applicants are suited to individualized and total nursing care and if they have the necessary commitment, knowledge, and skill?

The assumption that only A.A. or diploma graduates would be primary nurses or, for that matter, that only nurses with doctorates would be directors of nursing is misleading. Obviously, nursing needs to place people in the situation in which they belong and in which they desire to be. What is wrong with a B.S. graduate as a director of nursing or a nurse with a M.S. degree as a primary nurse? Would not this work under certain circumstances?

These questions are generally answered with the argument that in either case the individual's proposed talents would not be matched with the job. This point is debatable. People vary their jobs throughout their lifetimes, and it would be foolish to assume and be threatened by the fact that the wrong people (according to the degree they hold) are being placed in certain positions.

This one argument that usually culminates this discussion is our admission that the primary nurse role is indeed an attractive position and one to be envied, despite our degrees (which, as a matter of fact, span the field of possibilities in nursing).

How could you be sure you were truly evaluating primary nursing?

This question comes from those who are interested in our research and evaluation of primary nursing or who are skeptical about ever being able to measure anything in the hospital. It taps some major concerns about research in nursing and about evaluating any type of delivery of nursing care. In our studies, we went to great lengths to try to isolate the features of primary nursing and to measure them. We attempted to eliminate bias and to control for important factors. Primary nursing care units were compared with team nursing, functional nursing, and case method nursing units. Nursing units were compared before and after they had been converted to the primary nursing system. Nurses on primary nursing units were compared with nurses throughout the hospital with respect to salient characteristics, including age, experience in nursing, and experience working on their specific units, as well as according to the programs in nursing from which they had graduated. It was important to rule out these factors as causing the results obtained.

The sample of patients was randomly selected when possible. Groups of patients were matched according to sex, age, socioeconomic status, number of days hospitalized, number of times hospitalized, severity of illness, and stage of treatment. Care was taken to select days for gathering data that were considered "routine"; those days when patients or nurses may have been influenced by factors such as low census were avoided.

All these strategies were geared to eliminating uncertainty about what was measured. When certain extraneous variables that could affect the results of our research could be controlled, such as the personalities of nurses and perspectives of a certain kind of patient, as well as the fact that primary nursing care units were new and "special," more faith could be attached to our findings.

Our study met the criteria of a field experiment in every way except one: the units that would be primary nursing care units were not randomly selected. According to hospital administrators, this was not feasible. In each case, the hospital administrators had already selected one or more units to experiment with. They thought that certain units would benefit more by primary nursing than other units. For example, medical-surgical units with long-term patients would benefit from total patient care planning on a one-to-one relationship. In most cases, the obstetric, orthopedic, and neurosurgical units were not perceived as good candidates by administrators. Units rated high on the priority list were intensive care, coronary care, pediatrics, and general medical-surgical units with high proportions of terminally ill patients.

When we observed the neurosurgical unit and the obstetric unit, as well as all other units of a hospital benefiting from primary nursing care, we tended to agree with administrators for other reasons. First, on some of these units, patients were generally hospitalized for shorter periods of time. Second, clients were generally less amenable to answering questions and evaluating nursing care. In addition, these units would add a level of complexity in our analysis that would not be desirable for the pilot phase of research that we were in. We accepted these realities of our research field, which involves the ongoing operations of a hospital. Furthermore, we hoped that our explanations and predictions concerning outcomes of primary nursing care would be enhanced by the fact that we intended to collect our data from more than one hospital setting.

By evaluating data from more than one hospital, we were able to generalize our results to a greater degree. We were not required to conclude, "this is what we found in one hospital." Rather, we could conclude that this is what we found in hospitals in selected areas of the United States.

What are the areas that must be investigated—what about quality patient care?

This question is asked by many research- and evaluation-oriented nurses who are interested in further evaluation of primary nursing and who are up-to-date on current instruments for evaluation of quality patient care in a hospital setting.

There are many fertile areas of investigation. With regard to the satisfaction and accountability of primary nurses, more surveys need to be conducted to measure the turnover rate of nursing staff, the rate of errors on these units, and the degree of involvement of these nurses with patients. With regard to patient care, the following need further investigation: the degree that patients follow up on their treatment regimens, the rate of patient readmission, patients' levels of anxiety and knowledge about their care, and patients' sense of efficacy in influencing what happens to them. These areas focus on the outcomes of primary nursing for nurses and patients.

Another fruitful and important area needing further investigation, involves the changes that primary nursing implies in the organizational structure throughout the hospital. Roles and working relationships suggested by this system of nursing care need to be clarified. Additional data about how primary nursing affects supportive medical and hospital personnel need to be obtained systematically by research strategies.

Long-term data on any aspect of primary nursing are invaluable. The long-term effect of primary nursing on patients and on staff members is a vitally important issue. These kinds of studies will allow better description and prediction of overall effects of primary nursing care on patients, staff, and health care delivery. When the effects of primary nursing can be better described and predicted, then nurses will be provided with a sound basis for decision making about utilizing this nursing care modality.

INDEX